EVERYDAY BIOETHICS
Reflections on Bioethical Choices
in Daily Life

Giovanni Berlinguer

Policy, Politics, Health and Medicine Series
Vicente Navarro, Series Editor

BAYWOOD PUBLISHING COMPANY, INC.
Amityville, New York

Copyright © 2003 by Baywood Publishing Company, Inc., Amityville, New York

Baywood Publishing Company, Inc.

26 Austin Avenue
Amityville, NY 11701
(800) 638-7819
E-mail: baywood@baywood.com
Web site: baywood.com

Library of Congress Catalog Number: 2002018602
ISBN: 0-89503-225-2 (cloth)
ISBN: 0-89503-231-7 (paper)

Library of Congress Cataloging-in-Publication Data

Berlinguer, Giovanni.
    [Bioetica qutidiana. English]
    Everyday bioethics : reflections on bioethical choices in daily life / Giovanni Berlinguer.
        p. cm. - - (Policy, politics, health, and medicine series)
    Includes bibliographical references and index.
    ISBN 0-89503-225-2 (cloth) - - ISBN 0-89503-231-7 (pbk.)
      1. Medical ethics- -Miscellanea. 2. Bioethics- -Miscellanea. I. Title. II. Series.

R725.5 .B4513 2002
174'957- -dc21   2002018602

Preface

In these lines I would like to avoid summing up the theses of the book, for two reasons. One is a matter of substance: the ideas I present do not correspond to any systemic view and are often only provisional in nature. This is in part because the complexity of the moral choices deriving from scientific progress arouses in me (and, I think, in almost everyone) many and often conflicting thoughts. The other reason has a precautionary basis: I know from experience, as one who has sinned, that introductory outlines are often so extensive and exhaustive of the topic (and sometimes exhausting to the reader) as to give the reader the impression of having already read the book, or to dampen any enthusiasm to do so.

However, I owe my readers an explanation of the title I have chosen and of the path I followed in setting out my ideas. For some years now I have been addressing the problem of distinguishing between *everyday bioethics* and *frontier bioethics.*[1] My aim is to draw attention now focused almost exclusively on extreme cases— that is, on what was, prior to recent developments in biological science, infeasible and sometimes even inconceivable (such as medically assisted procreation, organ transplantation, artificial survival, guided genetic mutation, creation of new living species)—to the existence of another bioethics, less remote from everyday experience of ordinary people. Indeed, moral reflections on birth, on the relations between men and women and among different human populations, on the treatment of the sick, on death, on the interdependence of human beings and other living creatures—all have a very long history, almost as long as that of humanity itself. Today, wittingly or unwittingly, moral reflection guides the decisions of each ethnic or social group and of all individuals, even those furthest removed from the use or even the knowledge of the latest scientific breakthroughs. In other words, there are aspects of bioethics that have roots in the remote past, and there are ideas and values that daily permeate the minds and behaviors of all human beings and that deserve at least equal attention.

Additional stimuli over the past ten years have encouraged me to extend the investigation to other issues and, at the same time, to take a less schematic view

---

[1] I discussed this topic in a paper delivered at the Conference of Istituto Gramsci on "Questioni di vita: etica, scienza e diritto," March 11, 1988. The paper is published in the review *Rivista di teologia morale,* April–June 1988, pp. 63–768, and in the conference proceedings, *Bioetica,* edited by A. Di Meo and C. Mancina, pp. 5–18, Laterza, Bari, 1989.

of the distinction between everyday and frontier bioethics. A considerable contribution to this work has been provided by the exchange of ideas with Italian friends at home and with many others in international meetings and research. In these relations I have always perceived concerns and desires similar to my own. I detail these extremely useful encounters in the Afterword.

If the logical connections I make between the two fields of everyday bioethics and frontier bioethics sometimes appear somewhat forced, I must apologize to the reader; but I am increasingly convinced that the system of interrelations between the two is what gives rise to the most fruitful thinking about moral principles. On the other hand, it is precisely the boldest theories which tend to justify all high-risk biomedical technology, as proposed by bioethicists (proposals Alastair Campbell has likened to "bishops christening warships"), that encourage us to ponder these connections.

As I was correcting the final draft of this book, the heads of two influential nations, Tony Blair and Bill Clinton, opened the door to research on the use of stem cells. Stem cell research is deeply involved in creating the technologies whereby a given cell can be reproduced (cloned) and directed towards the development of new cells, capable of replacing tissue damaged by serious diseases such as Parkinson's and Alzheimer's. There is no doubt that these represent a concrete hope offered by science for the cure of serious and deadly diseases; the hope, that is, of cell cloning for a good cause. As soon as Blair's and Clinton's announcements were made public, a heated debate arose on the ethical problems raised by the use of stem cells of embryonic origin; the Parliament of the European Union announced a (highly restrictive) decision on September 7, 2000, and the House of Commons was called to decide on the matter in the United Kingdom. Public opinion, science, ethics, and politics are thus increasingly engaged in these topics, the complexities of which I have endeavored to analyze in Chapter 1.

The outcome of these developments, which lie midway between frontier and everyday bioethics, may be twofold. First, if legislation is enacted declaring, as in the official Roman Catholic moral code, that each embryo is a person, the decision seems inevitable that embryonic cells cannot be utilized, even those deriving from frozen embryos doomed to be destroyed, and not even for the purpose of saving from certain death individuals already born. But there is another likely logical consequence, concerning not only experimentation but also everyday life itself. The laws allowing abortion (under certain conditions) would have to be immediately abrogated, since taking the life of a "person" at a more advanced stage of growth would obviously be a more serious matter than using embryonic cells for therapeutic purposes. Abortion would again be within the purview of criminal proceedings, with women again forced to go underground and obstacles placed in the path of current reductions in abortion rates and future possible prevention (see Chapter 1).

The second outcome would pertain to cloning of cells or organisms, therapeutic or reproductive. Almost everyone has come out in favor of cell cloning for therapeutic purposes and against the cloning of human beings. Some people are afraid that the one practice will inevitably shade into the other. I do not share this fatalistic attitude. I am less worried by rash experimentation in this area than by the moral arguments put forward in its favor. The reproductive cloning of human beings—in other words, genetic predetermination—is being justified by the argument that, for all who are born, life is actually predetermined insofar as, instead of coming into the world as a kind of *tabula rasa,* they are born in a particular place, into a particular class, into a particular family, and to particular parents. My immediate reaction is not to deny the argument, which survives and flourishes, but to push it to its logical extreme. It could be said that all who come into this world today, anywhere, although born unique and singular, run a very serious risk of being strongly "standardized," with their ideas and behaviors beveled down to conform to those of other individuals. Thus they run the risk of becoming cultural and moral clones, cast in the same mold as so many others. On this basis it could indeed be argued, as a logical conclusion to this line of thinking, that there is no reason why genetic cloning should not be allowed. Otherwise, it could—and, indeed, must—be concluded that human freedom must prevail over all limits and obstacles, whether due to social injustice, the manipulation of minds, or genetic predetermination.

Table of Contents

CHAPTER 1

Procreation and Birth

PROCREATION AS FREE CHOICE

Although the expression "epoch-making" has been abundantly used and abused, especially during the transition from the second to the third millennium, it appropriately defines the changes in the field of human reproduction that began in the twentieth century. The advent of reproductive technology is one aspect of the changes in this field, changes that, indeed, moved the frontiers of science. These changes have a bearing on the daily life of a large number of human beings, affording the possibility of consciously regulating births and thus modifying the demographic situation: the demographic transition that began in the developed countries is now widespread and has begun to affect both birth and death rates.

So far, the use of reproductive technology has remained comparatively limited, and there is thus still no strong and widespread connection at a practical level between the technology and the demographic changes. On the other hand, ethical considerations have begun to present themselves. Although the moral issues emerging from the many changes vary, taken together they have given rise to a need to reflect on the beginning of human life. The depth of these changes has shaken many certainties and led to heated debate. This is only to be expected, because recognizing procreation as a free choice was a major component of the revolution in the relations between men and women, perhaps the most profound and longest lasting of the revolutionary changes that occurred in the twentieth century.

The freedom to procreate and, together with this, the freedom for children to thrive after birth are historical constructions typical of our times. In the past, unremitting procreation from puberty to menopause (which women rarely reached, owing to the incidence of early death) had been one of the major obstacles to women's full attainment of the status of multidimensional human beings.

In his *History of Women's Bodies,* Edward Shorter emphasizes that, in the past, women were "victims of nature," that is, of serious female-specific diseases, of sexual relations subordinated to male desire, and of the obligation of looking after at least half a dozen children (1). Only in the twentieth century were these difficulties reduced. This reduction made a substantial contribution, together with the civil and social struggles of their gender, to breaking what John Stuart Mill called the "subjection of women," which he compared to a widespread form of slavery (2). Furthermore, until the twentieth century, infant mortality had always been high (for the Italian poet Giacomo Leopardi this was the first sign of human destiny: "man struggles to be born / and his birth is a risk of dying"), and half of newborns died before the age of five. This was the price paid in terms of longevity, quality of life, and substantial freedom when the demographic dynamics were characterized by high birth rate and high mortality. These images from the past can be used to measure the progress made and to evaluate the limits to the spread of that progress in places, in classes, in ethnic groups, and in individuals living on the planet today.

FREEDOM, DUTIES, AND RIGHTS
OF PROCREATION

Freedom to procreate has increasingly implied both the theoretical and the practical rejection of ideas based on the conception of procreation as an obligation deriving from natural laws, political coercions, or religious precepts. The Catholic Church in particular has considerably changed its views on sexuality. Sexual intercourse between husband and wife, which in canon law had only two acknowledged purposes—*procreatio* and *remedium concupiscentiae*—after John XXIII and Vatican Council II was viewed not only as the duty to procreate but also as the expression of *bonum coniugium* deriving from the natural desire of man and woman. What has not changed is the criticism of birth control. The encyclicals *Casti connubi* and (later) *Humanae vitae* condemned in sexual intercourse "any act that . . . is aimed at or is a means for rendering procreation impossible" (3). Any act; yet couples may refrain from sexual intercourse during the woman's fertile periods by employing what is known as the "natural method" of birth control.

I shall not dwell on the theological justifications for this distinction (in this connection, see 4) but rather on the consequences of the directives it attempted to impose. The most obvious is that most Catholics almost always ignore these rules, often with the approval or tolerance of their ministers. Implicit sanction thus gave rise to a double moral standard: one preached and the other practiced. According to a survey conducted by the Italian Episcopal Conference in 1995, 70 percent of practicing Catholics do not accept the distinction between "natural" and "artificial" contraception, and only 15 percent obey the Church's rules on this matter.

These findings pertain essentially to the relationship between believers and their faith. Others also may be troubled, at the practical and moral level, by the insistent campaign carried out against the so-called "artificial" method, insofar as it increases the number of unwanted pregnancies and thus unwittingly encourages the practice of abortion. And it is of interest to everyone that, in the face of the danger of sexually transmitted diseases such as AIDS, the Church intervened, in Italy but even more vigorously in Argentina and several African countries, in order to prevent the state from promoting the use of condoms as a way of avoiding contagion. The cost in terms of human lives of the delays and obstacles deriving therefrom is difficult to quantify; what is certain, however, is that the cost was paid by both believers and nonbelievers.

What is clear, in any case, is that freedom in sexual relations and procreation (which includes also freedom *not* to procreate) also implies duties. The latter are to be viewed as responsibilities to one's dignity, to one's system of interpersonal relations, and, above all, to the as yet unborn. However, one controversial issue is whether there exists a *right* to procreation in addition to a *freedom*. Many (particularly women) doubt that the language of rights is the most appropriate language for dealing with matters such as procreation and birth, in which the predominant dimension is the relationship (both legal and, more importantly, affective) between the subjects, whose autonomy could be distorted by legislation and by state intervention. Then again, on the juridical plane, to shape a fully enforceable right is not always easy. This becomes obvious whenever the obstacle to procreation consists of sterility due to biological causes, such as anomalies or disease, at a time when there are both the means for preventing or treating such causes and a legal recognition of the right to health, as in, for example, article 32 of the Italian Constitution. But the question may arise whether assisted pro-creation, which works to circumvent sterility without removing the cause, repre-sents a right, and if so, for whom and under what conditions.

COMPULSORY AND INDUCED STERILIZATION

Despite the doubts about procreative rights, a broad consensus exists that to be arbitrarily deprived of such a right is unacceptable. Nevertheless, this has happened several times in history, even in the twentieth century, using medical means, for political or ideological reasons and even on humanitarian grounds—but mainly for selective purposes. Within the framework of policies to restrict the numbers of migrants from southern and eastern Europe to the United States, for example, by the late 1920s "two dozen states had approved as lawful the eugenic sterilization of mental patients. These laws were declared constitutional in 1927, in the Supreme Court decision in the *Buck v. Bell* case, which was explained by Judge Oliver Wendell Holmes on the grounds that 'three generations of imbeciles are enough' " (5).

Even more sensational cases occurred simultaneously in Germany, even before the advent of Nazism, involving the sterilization of handicapped and mentally deficient persons, under pressure from the wave of eugenics theory based on Galton's idea that it was useful to eliminate "undesirables" in order to improve the species. After Hitler came to power, sterilization was extended and became an integral part of Nazi racial programs. According to the ideologist H. W. Krantz, such programs had to be combined with the destiny of a "multitude of misfits, as many as one million, whose hereditary predisposition can be eradicated only through their elimination from the reproductive process" (6, cited in 7). After the fall of Nazism, the widespread indignation aroused by these practices appeared to have swept them away in all democratic countries. In actual fact, they continued silently in many parts of the world until, in 1997, the news was published that in Sweden (as well as in Austria, Norway, Denmark, the United States, and elsewhere even later), from 1946 to 1976, women who were carriers of disabilities or "the poor of mixed race" or the scholastically retarded continued to be sterilized.

Sometimes these practices were justified on the grounds of "their advantages": to avoid burdening these women with procreative responsibilities. However, compulsory intervention—sometimes concealed behind an unlikely consent as well as being directed in a discriminatory fashion only towards women (cases of male sterilization without consent being extremely rare)—runs counter to two fundamental acquired rights. One of these is the right of all human beings to the integrity of their own bodies. The other is the right to employ alternative methods of birth control free of fear of permanent impairment, a right that, thanks to scientific progress, is now available for the very rare cases in which preventing procreation is necessary.

In Italy, the National Bioethics Committee (CNB) has expressed a strongly critical opinion on "nonvoluntary sterilization" (8), citing also article 2 of the European Bioethical Convention, according to which "the interest and welfare of the human being must take priority over the interest of society and science." In addition to its negative opinion of eugenic sterilization, which it criticized for giving rise to "discrimination among the citizens, which is inadmissible in a state of law," the CNB has also criticized two other practices.

One is *penal sterilization,* that is, sterilization of those guilty of sexual offenses. It has no scientific justification at the therapeutic level and is not effective in preventing relapses, because violence, even if one considers it innate or irrepressible, can always be channeled in other directions. On the ethical-juridical plane, "it can barely conceal the primitive logic of juridical retaliation that underlies it." The absence of justification on theoretical or practical grounds is sufficient to refute the argument often advanced in the United States that, as capital punishment is appropriate for murder, so too are less serious corporal punishments such as sterilization appropriate for sexual violence. It may be added that, at this rate, the introduction of *lex talionis,* the law of retaliation, is only one step away.

The other practice is *demographic sterilization,* carried out in the name of population control. Compared with the pro-natalist coercion in vogue in Italy and Germany between the two World Wars, and later in several communist countries, demographic sterilization represents an opposite, anti-natalist coercion. The Italian CNB criticizes this procedure on moral grounds and adds a perspective based on experience: the facts have shown that "the declining birth rate is not the result of compulsory sterilization campaigns but of experiences of social modernization."

While I share many of the opinions represented in the CNB's remarks, which are common to many critical treatments of compulsory sterilization, I must express my disagreement with what the CNB considers *the fundamental ethical principle* on which to reject the various hypotheses: "the principle of the intangibility of the body, which should render illegitimate any intervention on it." I believe that this principle has been amply superseded by many beneficial techniques, starting with grafts and prostheses, and that we should avoid confusing the protection of the body and its intangibility, as, in other cases, we should avoid confusing its availability and its use as a commodity. The confusion of *protection* and *intangibility* could be detrimental to personal autonomy, which is precisely the value degraded by compulsory sterilization.

Among the many categories of sterilization subjected to critical review, that of *induced sterilization* is often neglected—that is, sterilization that appears to be voluntary but is actually coerced, as in cases of women who must accept sterilization in order to gain admission to a workplace or to avoid being marginalized or stigmatized. There are many established (and other concealed) cases of companies that have made employment contingent upon the demonstrated sterility of the candidate. I shall return to this topic in Chapter 3 with reference to ethical problems in the workplace. Italy's CNB has criticized the various cases of induced sterilization in the name of the substantive and not just the formal nature of autonomy: "Wherever pressure is exerted against essential aspects of a person's dignity and autonomy, it is impossible to assume a generalized sufficient level of freedom, which would demand a structure of the personality and of the resources which cannot be taken for granted, not even in the case of statistical majorities" (8, p. 26). In other words, it is the procreative freedom of those who are least able to withstand unlawful pressure that is in most need of protection.

STERILITY:
BIOPATHOLOGICAL, SOCIAL, AND CULTURAL

All cases are not equal, but the pressures applied to induce or impose the acceptance of sterilization are to a certain extent connected with factors restricting procreative freedom in general. They have not been sufficiently analyzed or opposed, and so Italian statistics in this area may be particularly interesting. Italy shares with Spain the lowest fertility rate in the world. The average number of children per woman is 1.17 for Spain and 1.18 for Italy, while it fluctuates between 1.50 and 1.80 in central and northern Europe. These indexes are almost certainly the lowest ever recorded in the world, in the history of our species, in "normal" periods—that is, excluding times of war, famine, pandemics, and other catastrophic events.

I shall not say whether this is good or evil. It is difficult to demonstrate that a community is happier under conditions of higher or lower birth rate, or that children grow up better if they are an only child or have brothers and sisters. Nor do I wish to subscribe to critical arguments outside the field of procreative choice that are based on moral judgments or social evaluations and are as categorical as they are unwarranted. I shall merely mention two arguments. One refers to the risk of ethnic and cultural contamination due to the higher birth rate of immigrants. This ignores or diminishes immigrants' rights and a society's advantages deriving from integration. The other argument criticizes the low procreation rate as being detrimental to the future contributions to pension funds. It ignores the existence of unemployment, which involves 10 to 20 percent of young people in Italy and Spain. If there were no jobless youth, existing and future pensions would be less exposed to risk, young people would probably marry earlier, and married couples would give less anxious answers to the question: "A child? And what will he do when he grows up?"

I shall not dwell on these topics, which, although stimulating political and social reflection, may deviate from bioethical analysis. In this field, again starting from the value of procreative freedom, there are many factors, among the choices acknowledged to be free, that prevent, hinder, penalize, or discourage precisely the choice to procreate. Among the subjective impediments associated with the "structure of the personality," which includes both mind and body, there is above all the increase in sterility of biopathological origin. A large body of research confirms this tendency, despite Niels Shakkebeak's argument (made in 1992) that, at the global level, a claimed mean reduction of 50 percent in men's sperm count between 1938 and 1991 could not be fully confirmed and is unlikely ever to be demonstrated (cited in 9). However, extensive documentation exists on the adverse effects of a number of environmental and workplace toxic agents on male and female fertility, and it is probable that men would have greater fertility if they stopped smoking, reduced body weight so as not to overheat the testicles, drank less alcohol and caffeine, and did not ingest hormones that may become testosterone. Also, the decision to shift parenthood to later in life is a factor that can increase a couple's relative sterility.

On the bioethical plane, as for all pathological conditions it is not possible to attribute a negative moral value to all cases of sterility (although, in the past and even now, sterility has been considered a stigma or fault, especially in women), because this condition may be due to anomalies or pathologies that are still unknown or nonmodifiable. Sterility takes on a negative moral significance when it represents a damage to the one sterilized, and an assumption of responsibility whenever an opportunity for preventive or curative action is not taken. This "sin of omission," which also represents the negation of procreative equal opportunity, involves not only medical intervention addressed to individuals but also an inadequacy of scientific research, imposed modification of personal behavior, and an absence of actions that might be taken to rehabilitate the (workplace and non-workplace) environment by controlling and reducing the factors affecting biopathological sterility.

Less obvious in this context is the increase in what might be termed social and cultural sterility. I shall not dwell on the psychological reasons or the multiple fears that lead to a reduction in procreation. They warrant attention and respect, except when they are reduced to criticism of so-called "female hedonism." I am not referring here to the numerous sociological studies on the personal behavior of the individual and the couple or to the understandable concerns linked to the idea of bringing children into this world (10). The research conducted in these fields is of great scientific and practical interest but does not explain the anomaly of Italy's birth rate. Similar conditions exist in countries with higher fertility rates, such as France and the United States. An analysis of the peculiar Italian (and Spanish) situation, which is deeply rooted in cultural and religious tradition, reveals two aspects: (a) a more difficult relationship between work and the female condition and (b) distortions in the welfare state. These attributes place Italy at a considerable distance from the rest of Europe in the area of equal opportunity of procreation. And at the personal level, procreation often becomes a joy accompanied by one or more punishments; the latter may be due to reduced incomes, shortcomings in social services, and the many difficulties encountered by the working woman.

Sometime declining birth rates are attributed to the increase in the number of women who work. However, this is confirmed neither by historical evidence nor by a comparative study of different countries. The truth is that, in response to the irreversible process, positive for both women and men, of women's freedom and emancipation, some nations have adopted welfare policies (work + support + services) designed to encourage this process, while others have not. These differences have been extensively documented and analyzed by Vicente Navarro, who reached the following conclusion: "The solution to low fertility and low participation by women in the labor market must be based on a growth in the services sector and, in particular, in personal and welfare services. The latter, while supporting the woman in her household matters, facilitate her integration in the workplace and at the same time extend the labor offer, satisfying her desire for greater autonomy" (11). The least that can be done to preserve the principle of autonomy for individuals and couples making procreative decisions—indeed, to make this principle available to all—is to "remove the penalties imposed on couples wanting to have children . . . even without waiting for the final results of a difficult debate of uncertain outcome as to what kind of balance there must, or rather ought to, be between population, resources and development" (12).

Only recently has Italy begun to move in this direction. Some progress has been made, although much too slowly, in the most important "service" on which equal opportunity for women to work, to procreate, and to lead lives of their own depends: the moral attitude and the personal commitment of men to share both household chores and the responsibility for raising children.

EQUITY FOR THE BORN CHILD

In bioethical debate, the concept of *equality* justly tends to be replaced by that of *equity*. The former, although retaining the driving force of justice it received from the French Revolution (combined with *liberté* and *fraternité*), often has been used to justify a tendency towards uniformity, to deny the value represented by the differences among individuals, genders, peoples. Its opposite—inequality—is still valid as a measure of the often enormous and growing differences in the human condition throughout the world. However, it does not tell us everything. It does not allow any clear-cut distinction (for instance, in quality of health) between what is due to natural conditions or free behavior and what depends on social and educational factors and thus requires moral evaluations of good and evil, right and wrong.

Evaluations based on the concept of equity, on the other hand, involve making a separate analysis of the causes, including human omissions and actions capable of increasing or reducing unfair differences, and taking into account not only access to but also acquisition of capabilities needed to attain a freely chosen goal. This view of equity implies a moral judgment that, in the field of procreation and childbirth, cannot have as its sole issue (as is often the case in the bioethical debate) the subjects and the modes of procreation or the status of embryos. At least equal attention must be devoted to the destiny of born children. That destiny is not just a matter of chance; it is strongly influenced by the conditions in which children will live, starting from their actual prospects of survival (see, e.g., 13).

Geographic differences in infant mortality (measured in number of deaths during the first year of life per thousand births) are very large, and tend to increase. In the U.N. report *Human Development 1999*, 174 world nations are classified according to a "human development index" (at last reference is not made exclusively to the economy!) based on three interrelated indicators: income, education, and health (14).The mean infant mortality of the 45 countries with the "highest human development" in 1970 was 25 per thousand, a number that dropped by more than two-thirds to 7 per thousand by 1997. The "low human development" countries had a rate of 147 per thousand in 1970 and 106 per thousand in 1997, a reduction of less than one-third. The differences, therefore, have tended to increase. After 27 years of spectacular progress in medicine and hygiene, many countries have benefited only minimally; others, not at all. Concrete examples at the lower end of the scale are Sierra Leone (from 206 per thousand in 1970 to 182 per thousand in 1997) and Nigeria (191 per thousand in 1970 and again in 1997). Conversely, in such countries as Sweden, Norway, Finland, and Japan, the index dropped to 4 per thousand births—that is to say, following the prevention and treatment measures taken in these countries, the probability of death during the first year of life is today *50 times less* than in Sierra Leone and Nigeria. Such figures are also an indicator of social equity, because the four deaths of newborns per thousand births, rather than representing instances of improvidence or lack of care, suggest causes due to chance or to still-incurable fetal pathologies. The protective measures taken in the countries with the lowest child mortality figures are such that, whatever the place, the family, or the class into which a child is born, its chances of survival are practically the same as those of any other child born in that country. Elsewhere, to a greater or lesser degree, an unnatural, socially determined selection prevails.

Or, as is particularly the case in several Asian countries (but not only in there), the selection is gender determined. Figures revealing the unnatural imbalance in population between males and females, adjusted for genetic and environmental risk and calculated for the demographic trends of the whole twentieth century, are summed up in the dramatic phrase "a hundred million missing women." How many women are missing? The imbalance in favor of males as documented by censuses has been calculated using two different methods: one concludes that there are 44 million missing women in China, 37 million in India, and a total of 100 million in the world; the other, 29 million in China, 23 million in India, and 60 million in the world. These data, which show that cultural and social discrimination succeed in overturning women's biological superiority (from the first few days of life, survival of females is greater, under normal conditions, than that of males), were reported by Amartya Sen (15). Based on a large body of evidence, he attributes to traditional values and economic interests practices that include the neglect of female children in health care, fewer female admissions in hospitals, inferior female diet, and higher female infant mortality, both natural and induced. One reason for the lower female population in China, he adds, is the constraint of being allowed only one child. To show that this tendency can be reversed, he reports the example of the state of Kerala, in India, where the situation was changed by means of education and health care for all and recognition of the value of women's rights and their contributions to the economy and to the life of the community. He concludes that the missing women "may be rescuable after all, by public policy."

Frontier bioethics today includes discussions of whether it is morally legitimate, as is now possible with assisted procreation, to choose the unborn child's sex. Daily experience tells us that 60 to 100 million women have disappeared from statistics (and from life) as a result of selective processes favoring males right from birth. This selection can now be done even earlier. Medical technology now allows us to know the sex of the unborn child, and technology (diagnosis and abortion) can be used to support atavistic customs to replace or supplement infanticide, denial of care, and other forms of discrimination that have led to the tremendous gender imbalance. The recognition of equal rights and opportunities for women, which has arisen almost everywhere in recent decades, has reduced these practices. The decisions of the Indian government to pay a 500 rupee endowment to mothers who give birth to (and accept) a female newborn and its attempt to restrict the use of ultrasound examination are laudable, but they do not seem sufficient to eliminate gender-based selection. Such selection is based on persistent local concepts, interests, and customs as well as on the guilty silence of the rest of the world.

I have spoken of social and gender selection. What about natural selection? It still exists, starting with the fact that a large number of fertilized ova do not successfully implant in the uterus, and many embryos do not survive because they are unsuitable for development. In these cases almost no practical remedy exists, nor any desire to save them, nor any moral concern. However, natural selection has been reduced considerably, particularly in the subsequent stages of life. Prevention and care during and after pregnancy today guarantee the survival of fetuses that ten years ago (and, to an even greater extent, a hundred years ago) would have been ineluctably doomed to die.

Demographers and philosophers wonder about the consequences of this state of affairs, and some regret is voiced from time to time over the reduced role of natural selection in the world today. The debate has been analyzed by Andrea Furcht (16), starting from the fears emerging in British culture and in various eugenic schools of thought between the nineteenth and twentieth centuries and continuing up to the present-day observations of Jacques Monod. Monod expressed concern and alarm over the fact that, in modern societies, "selection has been abolished. At least, there is no longer anything 'natural' about it in the Darwinian sense of the term" (17). And what is more, he added, "in even recent times, even in 'advanced' societies, the elimination of the physically and mentally weaker individuals was automatic and cruel. The majority did not live beyond puberty. Nowadays, many of these genetically diseased persons live long enough to reproduce. . . . The non-selective or, rather, reverse-selective conditions that prevail in the advanced societies are to some extent a danger to the species."

When commenting on these assertions, Furcht begins by asking, "How many tears should be shed over the end of natural selection?"—especially because the path through history of natural selection "is paved with blood and suffering." Other researchers observe that selective pressure is today offset by other factors that tend to increase selection, such as pathogenic agents that used to be isolated and are now widespread and the increase in environmental factors that produce genetic mutations (18, cited in 16). Then there is the greater size and greater mobility of the population, compared with preceding societies, which reduces the probability of the meeting of genes responsible for diseases of a recessive nature; at the limit of this scattering of genes, this kind of disease could even disappear. It is thus possible to be more complacent about the danger of the gradual degeneration of our species that Monod considered inevitable, although he situated it some 10 or 15 generations hence. On the other hand, we ought to be concerned about implicit re-proposals of selective ideas that might lead to omission of possible action in support of weaker individuals, individuals doomed to die if not helped. Neither utilitarian theories nor those based on the intrinsic value of every human life can justify even passive selection in the name of an alleged advantage for the species.

THE SUBJECTS OF ASSISTED PROCREATION

Probably the most morally controversial issues concerning childbirth today are related to medically assisted procreation. Even though it is often isolated from the general context of procreation and childbirth, a more detailed examination of this bioethical topic—situated at the cutting edge of biomedicine, intrinsically extremely complex, morally involving, and bound up with difficult political decisions—may also allow the values and choices made every day, by everyone in the field of procreation, to be specified more clearly.

A preliminary question is whether in procreation (as in any field of bioethics) a different moral evaluation should be made between *natural* and *artificial*. Assisted procreation consists typically of a correction of "nature's mistakes" and thus is taken to represent a completion of human potentialities. The hostility towards assisted procreation is fed by a static conception of the relationship between nature and science. Science and technologies can increase human choices and human freedom, but we must not underestimate the preoccupation with the separation of assisted reproduction from human experiences such as desire, sexuality, love, parenthood, and childhood, as well as the dependence on a highly invasive medicine in which priority is given to quick technical remedies, sometimes concealing the relative risks and drawbacks as well as the failures.

For instance, one recently introduced procedure is the use of a single spermatozoon to fertilize an ovum in vitro. Normally, millions of spermatozoa are contained in each ejaculation and must compete to reach the ovum. Thus there is a selective process that in vitro fertilization abolishes without any prior assessment of the consequences. One extreme example of what the *Lancet* called "science versus clinical adventurism" (19) uses spermatids for fertilization in cases of azoospermy (the absence of spermatozoa in the seminal fluid). Spermatids are immature forms that are extracted directly from the spermatic ducts; their DNA is frequently found to be altered. Although there is no unanimous consensus on the facts, I consider the concluding analysis in the *Lancet* article to be appropriate (19, p. 517):

> The rapid advances in reproductive technology are driven not only by scientific curiosity and capabilities, but also by profit, and by patients' demand. These factors explain why new reproductive techniques have been adopted so rapidly—more so than in other medical specialties—without rigorous studies and solid evidence of long-term safety. Ironically, because the errors have implications for the health of future generations, there is no other medical specialty in which mistakes could have such dire consequences for practitioners and for the children so conceived.

These predictions of hypothetical but frightening consequences are based on existing documentation of children born by means of medically assisted procreation: here we find a higher frequency of twin, and thus premature, births; an increase in newborns with lower than normal weight; increased perinatal mortality and malformations; and a greater need for intensive care. Medically assisted procreation is also associated with the suffering of many women subjected to "procreative over-medication," which abuses their bodies and souls. These facts and uncertainties call for more thorough research, a curtailing of the speed with which science moves from acquiring knowledge to applying it, a more intense use of the principle of precaution, and a medical ethics that is more respectful of human rights. But they certainly do not cancel out the fact that the vast majority of the "children of science" are born healthy and live as happily as the "children of nature," and that they are the result of a free choice made by their parents.

Are there any limits to this freedom? Some limits may arise out of choices made according to conscience. Those who think, for example, that "the desire of the individual cannot detract from the value of 'biological derivation,' which is . . . a clear indication of God's intentions as written into biological reality" (20), a reality sanctified by marriage, may well reject fertilization using a donor's semen, in the procedure known as "heterology"—a term used in biology to refer to cross-breeding between different species! Those who instead think that in addition to biological derivation—and even more important than this, in the opinion of some—recognition must be given to affective filiation, may justly consider assisted procreation to be morally acceptable when there is no other alternative for having a child.

I am speaking of two different tendencies based on individual conscience. However, the laws must reflect and, to some extent, guide a pluralistic society based on the inseparable combination of freedom and responsibility and, thus, must not impose constraints that have no demonstrable rational foundation, such as the idea that direct genetic derivation from both legal parents is the only way to have happy children. The state cannot merely declare that what biomedical science does is lawful, nor is it possible to avoid the issue through tacit or explicit acknowledgment of the autonomous "moral communities" recorded by H. T. Engelhardt (21). If we mean to create rules designed to favor civil coexistence and the respect of individuals, the starting point must be that two different types of subject are involved in assisted procreation: those who choose to be involved and the yet unborn. There is a widespread tendency to suggest that, while recognizing the legitimate and normally converging values of both subjects, priority should be given to the needs of the child yet to be born.

The arguments in favor of the latter thesis frequently appeal to solidarism, to the primacy of the "rights of the weaker." A restrictive interpretation of the theory of rights, however, states that only those who exist (and according to some, only those who have awareness) can claim rights, not those who do not yet exist. This interpretation may, however, be refuted on the basis of the principle of duty that underpins Kantian moral philosophy: I must behave "in such a way as to want my principle to become a universal law" (22). When extended to human conception

(23), this principle implies a commitment by the parents to the quality of life of the yet to be born. However, the relationship with children, according to Jonas, represents "*one* case (which deeply moves the observer) of an elementary *non-reciprocal* responsibility and obligation, which is recognized and practiced spontaneously" (24). The motivation for this behavior is not the expectation that, in one's old age, one may be compensated for the love and attention dispensed to one's children. The attitude towards them is unconditional: "This is the only example in *nature* of a totally altruistic behavior," Jonas writes. "Indeed, it is this relationship, linked to the biological event of reproduction and *not* the relationship between independent adults (from which derives the idea of reciprocal rights and duties), that underlies the idea of responsibility as such."

On a practical plane, the case furthest away from this moral dimension is probably that of the child in the United States who, at birth, was lawfully an orphan of five parents, all still alive. The explanation is a simple one. Two of them (parents 1 and 2), who originated the procreative decision, were a sterile couple who wanted a child. They applied to a semen and ovum bank to receive from "donors" (parents 3 and 4) the male and female gametes required and, after fertilization in vitro had taken place, contracted out the pregnancy to a "surrogate mother" (parent 5). Just prior to the birth, however, parents 1 and 2 separated and declared they no longer intended to accept a child; parent 5, after giving birth and thus honoring her contract, declared she had no intention of keeping the newborn; while parents 3 and 4 had long since disappeared into anonymity. Everything in order, except for the newborn's prospects. As well as this extreme case, numerous other variants are extensively reported in the media in which the "completely altruistic behavior" to which the criterion of responsibility cited by Jonas refers is ridden over roughshod or disregarded.

For these reasons there is a need more or less everywhere for moral rules, in some cases accompanied by juridical norms. Italy's National Bioethics Committee, according to its statement of June 17, 1994, had found a substantial consensus among all its members, from different disciplines and cultural schools of thought, on the guidelines to be adopted in allowing access to medically assisted procreation (25):

> The well-being of the child to be born must be considered the central reference criterion in the evaluation of the various opinions on procreation. This criterion suggests that, as a general rule, the best condition in which a child may be born is that of having been conceived and brought up by an adult couple of different sexes, either a married couple or one that is at least stably united by a communion of life and love. It is also preferable that this couple should be of a potentially fertile age, even though, for various reasons, it may actually be affected by infertility. It is also a fundamental principle that the birth of a human being must be the result of an explicit shouldering of responsibility—with all juridical implications—by those demanding recourse to assisted procreation. The public institutions must therefore make every

effort to make those benefiting from assisted procreation aware of their responsibilities and to ascertain the seriousness of the commitment they thereby undertake.

EQUAL OPPORTUNITIES AND THE IDENTITY OF THE CHILD TO BE BORN

Almost all the European countries have passed legislation more or less in keeping with these guidelines. Italy, on the other hand, has moved away from them: first, until 1999, through its long legislative silence; and then by proposing bills that, instead of ensuring the general consensus required in such a delicate field of public action, deeply split the country along lines of political speculation and explicit ideology. It is paradoxical that such strongly restrictive regulations should be proposed after the legislative bodies had for so long obstructed the introduction of any regulations at all and after ignoring *de facto* and allowing *de jure* all kinds of abuse—including the possibility for a husband, after explicitly accepting his wife's fertilization with a donor's semen, to refuse to recognize the child after birth. I do not know whether the principal foundation for this hostility is the hypocritical criterion that it is better to ignore a sin than to approve of it by law or the idea (translated into a court decision by the Cremona magistrate in 1994; 26) that "heterologous" insemination is to be deemed "genetic adultery." The Supreme Court (*Corte Costituzionale*) later decided that this decision was unlawful.

A further consequence of the refusal to legislate is the persistent absence of elementary technical, scientific, and legal guarantee regulations for centers providing assisted procreation services, regulations essential to ensuring that the beneficiaries enjoy equal safety, hygiene, and protection against abuse. These regulations have been proposed by various commissions and could have been adopted even by simple ministerial decree; however, they have always been blocked at the time of political decision. The CNB has also contributed to blocking them, claiming that it was necessary to establish first the moral criteria and then the technical, safety, and legal regulations.

I have mentioned the long legislative silence in Italy. To tell the truth, one regulation was actually introduced with unusual timeliness, on March 1, 1985. An examination of this regulation could lead us to a criterion that should be essential in evaluating regulatory activity in the field of medically assisted procreation—that of equality of opportunity. I refer to the discriminatory element contained in the only regulation that, although with the low juridical profile of a ministerial circular, sees rigorous application. The circular bears the signature of Costante Degan, minister for health at the time, and is entitled "Limits and Conditions of Legitimacy of Artificial Insemination Service within the National Health Service" (see 27). It bans "heterologous" insemination in the public health services on the basis that "the essential foundation of the relationship of filiation is that of biological derivation" and that "only techniques involving the use of the couple's gametes will allow their desire to be realized without raising doubts as to the paternity and maternity of the unborn child."

It is debatable whether this circular represents a protection or an abuse. What is undeniable is that, being limited to the public health service and not making provision for any bans, regulations, or control in private medicine, it has created a dual path: it allows a remedy for many types of sterility to be obtained only by those able to pay for it. To my knowledge, nowhere in the bioethical field in Italy or other European countries are there any such regulations aimed at officially introducing a "double standard." The only similarity is with the prevailing trend in the United States, where restrictive regulations apply in many fields of scientific research and biomedicine to institutions benefiting from federal funds, while those using private funds are not subject to such regulation. The main difference is that in Italy the double standard is based on ideology, while in the United States it is based on the market.

On the procreation market, gametes are bought and sold and the uterus is for hire. On October 24, 1999, high-sounding headlines appeared in the dailies, such as: "Models' Ova Auctioned over Internet" (*Corriere della sera*); "Want to Have a Child with a Top Model? With Internet You Can" (*l'Unità*); "AAA Ova for Sale on Internet for Children Guaranteed Beautiful" (*La Repubblica*); and on October 26, "Everyone in the Queue for Superkids" (*La Stampa*). The headlines were triggered by the announcement made on the Internet by Ron Harris, a Hollywood photographer, that he was auctioning the ova of supermodels. Comments inside and outside the United States were almost unanimously contemptuous, with occasional references to Hitlers "Lebensborn" mating houses, where beautiful Teutonic Aryans mated with SS officers to produce the finest specimens of the race. However, as is often the case nowadays, the Internet is only the tip of the iceberg; deep below, or else floating unseen on the surface, is a huge concealed mass of similar occurrences: hence, the indignant reaction to Karen Synesiu—who runs the misnamed "Ova Donation" agency, paying each "donor" $2,500 to $5,000 and offering the ova to her clients "describing their characteristics, and they make their choice"—seems quite out of place. She herself is part of a flourishing trade in sperm and eggs, accompanied by catalogs illustrating their quality and price, a trade that has been extensively documented (see 28, 29). While there are well-founded doubts about the procreative success of these choices (suggesting the possible aggravating circumstance of fraud), the moral intention is that of selling or buying a selective advantage, of predetermining the genetic characteristics of one's children, and of violating the principles of autonomy and equal opportunity for the future child.

In the case of "substitute mothers on commission," what is at stake, in the broad sense, is also the principle of human dignity. In very simple terms, this is based on the Kantian precept of "always considering man as an end, never only as a means," a standard incompatible with the marketing of the body. The voluntary act of "temporary donation of one's uterus," as has been done between women of the same family, is sometimes considered in a different moral light. In both cases, however, the principle of the preeminent subject being the child to be born has led to reflection on the depth of the relationship created with the pregnant woman during the intrauterine life and on the damage that may be caused by its abrupt cessation after the birth (30). This act "is in contradiction with the scientifically supported observation of decisive psychological exchanges between the pregnant woman and the fetus, as a result of which the subsequent separation can only be traumatic for both" (31). The analysis must not, however, be carried out only in terms of pathologies with preliminary case histories but not yet any undisputed epidemiological assessment. It must also be developed in relation to the child's personal identity, its construction of self, within a system of relations that may include several maternal figures, that may appear to its eyes complex and inexplicable, that are sometimes obscured by silences and lies.

One of the most controversial issues involving those born by "heterologous" procreation is related to their right to know who their genetic parents are. However, this issue does not concern only "test-tube babies." It also concerns adopted children, as it is not right to establish two different rules, giving some an opportunity that is denied others. This issue may apply also to other cases such as that of a child, even one born naturally to a legally married couple, who wants information about the family's history of genetically transmitted diseases or proneness thereto. These needs are part of the *right to know,* which is gradually extending in many fields as an expression of personal autonomy. In the case of medically assisted procreation, this right is offset by the practical consideration that, if it were possible to trace the semen (or ovum) donors, donations would cease to be available and, as an indirect consequence, a black market or a migration towards other countries for procreative services would arise. Concern over these possibilities (sometimes accompanied by *bioethical tourism* to neighboring countries, as in the case of Italians traveling to the United Kingdom before Italy's abortion law) arose in Sweden after it enacted laws allowing freedom of information regarding one's genetic parents. Experience has shown, however, that, after the withdrawal of many traditional, young, unmarried donors, numerous other adult ones, married and with children, offered their semen with the consent of their families.

TOWARDS THE PREVENTION OF ABORTION?

Abortion is the dark side of the reproductive functions. Dark, because it often comes about as a result of unknown causes or of tormented decisions. Dark, because it represents a negative conclusion to the procreative process. And dark because, whether it occurs through choice or tragic accident, abortion is a centuries-old scourge for fertile women. Abortion, which has rightly been called "a dilemma of our age" (32), until the mid twentieth century was hidden, emerging from the shadows only in cases of lethal consequence or criminal prosecution, usually for the woman. The first international congress that treated abortion as a global issue was held in the United States in 1967, after the feminist and civil rights movements, jurists and physicians, sociologists and legislators had shed light on the alarming dimensions of the problem and had begun to demand laws that, under certain circumstances, would allow legal abortion with the assistance of the health services. Since that time, abortion has become the subject of bitter controversy, of movements for and against, of philosophical reflection, and of laws proposed and often passed.

This recent history of abortion controversy includes Italy as well as other countries. As a deputy and rapporteur in the Chamber of Deputies, I participated in the long process that preceded passage of the bill named "Norme per la tutela sociale della maternità e sull'interruzione volontaria della gravidanza" (Norms for the social protection of maternity and on the voluntary interruption of pregnancy). The process lasted six years: from 1972 to 1976 and, after new elections, from 1976 until its final approval on May 18, 1978. I shall discuss the bioethics of abortion on the basis of the Italian experience, even if my point of view may legitimately be viewed as biased. However, it reflects, although perhaps in a distorted way, what was the broadest, longest, and most controversial bioethical debate ever to take place in Italy. That debate involved a confrontation between, not two, but many positions, and it brought to light the dilemmas that are still engaging philosophical analysis, public decisions, and the conscience of single individuals.

I shall not dwell on an analysis of the law, promulgated as law no. 194 in the *Gazzetta Ufficiale (Official Gazette)* of May 22, 1978 (33). We may begin with a question. Why, after it had been approved with a slight 52 percent majority in the Chamber of Deputies and 51 percent in the Senate, when two years later it was subjected to an abrogative referendum, called by the Christian Democratic Party, was the law confirmed by 68 percent of Italians (70 percent in Rome)? I think that a minority, among those who voted for confirmation, did so to register their approval of abortion as a symbol of women's freedom. The vast majority voted as they did because they considered abortion to be a symptom and an incarnation, the most widespread and hitherto the least understood, of the tragedies of women, of the iniquity, abuse, and violence that continue even today in many areas of life. A few wanted, by means of their vote, to give a moral approval of abortion. Many others considered that only by bringing the phenomenon out into the open, legalizing it, and providing assistance, would it be possible to begin limiting the damage and working on prevention.

The majority thus confirmed that, in view of previous experience and within certain conditions, it was right to eliminate previous references to penal legislation (even in terms of "unpunishable offense") and that, in these cases, the decision of whether or not an abortion should take place should be made by the woman rather than delegated to authority, whether physician or magistrate. Previous experience pointed to three clear conclusions: (*a*) penal sanctions drive the phenomenon underground, failing to eliminate the problem and only aggravating women's suffering; (*b*) lack of approved assistance creates unfair disparities, based on wealth and education, in both the quality of the operation and its outcome; and (*c*) bringing abortion out into the open is the only way to begin the work of eliminating the evils attendant on its practice.

The direct vote confirming the law was based on these experiences and, in practical terms, expressed confidence in the possibility of reducing both the number of abortions and the suffering resulting from them. It was not "pro-abortion." This vote was based on a distinction between the concept of legality, as an acknowledgment of a behavior that ought not to be liable to legal punishment, and that of morality, as a validation of the behavior as morally defensible. The positive evaluation of abortion on a moral plane disregards the fact that it represents the interruption of a life process in which the two gametes, male and female, are united to begin the development of a unique being. It is the tragic outcome of a conflict between, on the one hand, a human being in the process of formation and, on the other, a woman's own health, needs, and aspirations.

Not all observers agree with this evaluation. In the document *In Defense of the Right to Abortion*, published by the Consulta italiana di bioetica on October 19, 1993, for example, there are two aspects worth examining. One is the title itself, as there is a difference between "legal possibility" and "right," and law no. 194—which the document sets out to defend—opens up a possibility but does not sanction a right. The other is the definition of gestation. It is stated in the document that "Gestation, which begins with the implantation of the embryo in the uterus wall, is a biological process that belongs solely to the woman's body; it is the woman's body that makes possible the, albeit genetically determined, processes of differentiation and growth resulting from natural or artificial fertilization." I find this definition restrictive and questionable on ethical and scientific grounds. The use of the words "belongs" and "solely" effectively obscures the interactive nature of the growth process, which takes place between two subjects; and the word "biological" fails to encompass the psychological and affective components of a relationship whose importance, always empirically accepted, has now been confirmed by numerous scientific studies.

I began with law no. 194, of which I was the convinced rapporteur. I found myself subsequently perplexed and even anguished when the abortion figures in the first two years after the law's enactment were found to be high and even seemed to be increasing. Now, in view of the results obtained over time, I am a champion of the law's application in all its parts, especially those providing for prevention, which, for reasons I shall endeavor to explain, were the provisions most neglected. The law (like similar ones passed in Europe) may legitimately be criticized at the moral level as an acknowledgment and validation of abortion. It is also criticized at the practical level for two reasons: one is that legal abortion has not succeeded in eliminating illegal abortion; the other is that the effects of law no. 194 are comparatively insignificant in decreasing the number of legal abortions, arguing that if normal pregnancies decrease rapidly it is normal for abortions to decrease. The essential figures, coming out of the annual reports of the Ministry of Health, are the following. First, between 1982 and 1993 *legal abortions* decreased by 35.7 percent (i.e., by more than one-third), and between 1993 and 1994 by a further 5 percent. Second, the number of *illegal abortions,* as estimated by the Ministry of Health, was 350,000 before 1978 and dropped to 100,000 in 1983 and 52,000 in 1993 (i.e., about one-seventh the number prior to the passing of the law). Third, the *abortion rate,* expressed as the number of voluntary interruptions of pregnancy per thousand women aged between 15 and 45 years, decreased by 39 percent compared with 1982, and continues to decrease. Finally, the abortion rate as a function of the number of births (which represents the number of voluntary abortions per thousand live neonates and is, of these numbers, the most significant and the hardest to reduce) is now 273 per thousand, a reduction of 28.2 percent (i.e., more than one-quarter) compared with 1982, when it was 380 per thousand live neonates.

These data in no way influence the ethical debate on abortion, since ethics cannot be quantified. Even if there were only a single case, the conflict opposing a woman, as a living and autonomous person, to an embryo would still be agonizing. However, the above data lead us to a consideration that, while starting in the statistical realm, can move to the ethical. Because it has proved possible over two decades to reduce significantly the number of abortions, by between one-third and nearly one-half, depending on the indicators used, an ambitious goal could be proposed to reduce this number even further. In the space of a few generations, this universal drama that for thousands of years has brought torment and tragedy to women (and to unborn children) and has created such turmoil in human society could ultimately become a marginal phenomenon in developed societies. And tomorrow, though widening statistical gaps make the future harder to predict, perhaps in other areas of the world we will see alternatives to abortion increasingly embraced.

If this possibility exists, the question is, what ideas and what approach can accelerate the attainment of such a goal? There are obviously numerous possible answers; they are related to the female condition, to the relations between men and women and between the generations, to the value assigned to procreation and life, to the common consent that can be established for this objective, and to the social and ethical climate of our age. However, I believe the approach that can attract the widest consensus and lead to major results most quickly, and the one most directly linked to public ethics and its applications, is that of prevention.

This approach has two aspects, which, using terms borrowed from medicine (perhaps inappropriately), I would define as primary prevention and secondary prevention. The former consists above all of the regulation of conception, in responsible sexuality, in attempting to avoid the unwanted or unplanned pregnancy ending in abortion; the other consists of encouraging acceptance by means of solidarity and assistance. The first aspect acts by preventing pregnancy; the second is subsequent to fertilization and thus related to an ongoing process. An analysis of the Italian experience seems to indicate that the same culture that opposed law no. 194 opposed also the use of effective birth control, and therefore are responsible for the limited success of primary prevention. An important role in causing the shortcomings in secondary prevention was played by other subjects, those that insisted on a reductive interpretation of a woman's role, as though her liberation and emancipation could take place only if her maternal function was obscured. This view opposed as mutually exclusive the idea of the wholly liberated and fulfilled woman and the woman who was "only a mother," an interpretation that feminist movements have substantially corrected in recent years.

In the case of prevention, some thought should be given, even before any reference is made to the welfare and social services, to that complex of ethical concerns upon which John Paul II (I even dare to say, at long last) dwells in sections 58 and 59 of the Encyclical *Evangelium vitae* (34):

> It is true that in many cases the decision to abort takes on a dramatic and sorrowful nature for the mother, as the decision to rid herself of the fruit of conception is not taken for reasons of pure selfishness or convenience, but for the purpose of safeguarding a number of important values, such as one's own health or a dignified standard of living for the other members of the family. . . . The decisions concerning the child to be born are often made by other persons as well as the mother. Above all, the father of the child may be guilty, not only when he explicitly urges the woman to abort, but also when he indirectly encourages her decision in this sense because he has left her to face the problems of pregnancy alone.

Numerous other cases could be cited, even including those in which the woman is explicitly obliged to choose between pregnancy and keeping her job. In essence, while abortion has tended so far to be blamed mainly on the spread of immorality and the selfishness or hedonism of women, there are clearly other factors that encourage abortion and that must be tackled through the help and maturation of society as a whole. The laws, the services, the human solidarity are all complementary to this commitment.

Is it therefore necessary to change law no. 194? It is worth observing what the law itself states in this connection: in article 2.d it specifies that the tasks of the clinics (tasks that may be extended to any service) include providing information on the laws protecting working mothers, providing support at the level of local authorities and other structures, and contributing to "overcoming the causes that could lead the woman to terminate her pregnancy." During the parliamentary work, this article was reformulated at the request of Catholic deputies to emphasize the preventive function of the services and to change public perception of abortion practices by reaffirming the interest of the state in taking dissuasive (and certainly not coercive) action against the woman's decision to abort. Very little of all this has actually been implemented in practice. The needs of women and of the children to be born have often taken second place to the clash between ideologies and political factions, the obstacles placed in the path of the clinics and their medicalization, and, above all, the weakening of social ethics in Italy and elsewhere during the 1980s and 1990s.

Is it possible to start from the existing policies I have cited, or should we give priority to modifying the law? In my opinion, not only does the second option lead to a dead-end, but the very fact of giving it priority is a hindrance to prevention, which has the advantage of offering gradual rather than traumatic change, using a practical rather than an ideological approach. Prevention could have three effects: to accelerate the process of reducing abortions, provide a clearer perception of the benefits but also of the limits of the laws, and contribute to increased confidence when bringing children into the world.

EMERGING PROBLEMS: EXPERIMENTATION INVOLVING EMBRYOS

I hope (although I am not certain) that this norm-based analysis has made a clear statement of the complex bioethical issues relating to abortion. It might have been possible to employ other approaches and to obtain better results, starting from the subject—the woman, concerning whom feminist thinking has come up with illuminating ideas; the father, *semper ignotus* in ethical and social evaluations; the couple; the embryo—or else from the different opinions of philosophers and scientists. My general preference for taking as the basis of my analyses both facts and experience (professional and personal) was in this case heightened by my vision of an alliance in which science, law, and ethics use the common language of prevention to begin to solve the problem that abortion presents. Such a united approach would become even more effective should scientists at the cutting edge of biomedical science create new knowledge with practical applications, although questionable experiments involving human embryos and cloning are unlikely to help clarify these issues.

Besides its connection with abortion, the embryo has emerged as a topic of study and discussion in the field of medically assisted procreation, especially in relation to decisions about the number and destiny of embryos not intended for implantation in the uterus as well as the question of the legitimacy or illegitimacy of experiments on human embryos. The difficulty of reaching agreement and introducing uniform laws in this field is demonstrated by the fact that the European Bioethical Convention (35) promoted by the Council of Europe, which in many fields expresses a policy shared by its 41 member countries, does not mention medically assisted procreation and merely makes two references to the embryo, both in article 18. One states somewhat hypocritically that "wherever the law allows in vitro research on embryos, it must provide adequate protection for the embryo," as though research itself did not almost always imply profound alterations of the embryo. The other one, more precise in its language, affirms that "the creation of embryos for research purposes is not permitted." It imposes a just limit and should successfully avoid the extreme case of the creation of "embryo factories," although the question of whether it is legitimate in general to carry out experiments on embryos is eluded.

In the years that followed, the European Steering Committee on Bioethics (CDBI) endeavored to work out common definitions for these topics, which still proves a difficult task. The estimate, based on the preparatory work for a *Protocol on the Protection of Human Embryo and Fetus,* is that it will take one or two additional years (or more) to reach any conclusions. The list of chapter headings for the preliminary text is enough to show how difficult this is: "Definition of the Embryo and the Fetus" (it is proposed to consider the zygote, until it is implanted in the uterus, as an embryo; in all subsequent stages, a fetus); "Protection of the Embryo in Vitro"; "Choices of Persons Regarding Their 'Own' Embryos"; "Research on Embryos in Vitro"; "Research in Vivo on the Embryo, the Fetus, and the Woman"; "Fetal Therapy"; "Prenatal Diagnosis"; "Feto-Maternal Conflicts"; "Sampling of Embryonic and Fetal Cells and Tissues"; "Use of Embryonic and Fetal Tissues"; "Consensus."

My first impression on reading this text was of an excessive tendency to insist on detailed regulations that are difficult to enforce, almost always accompanied by exceptions allowed on the basis of national legislation. This impression is heightened by the *restricted* nature of the texts; that is, they are circulated among a small group of persons until after they have been approved. This practice clashes with, among other things, article 38 of the European Bioethical Convention itself: "The contracting parties assure that the fundamental questions raised by the developments of biology and medicine are the subject of a public debate in view, in particular, of the medical, social, economic, ethical, and juridical implications, and that their possible applications are subjected to appropriate consultations." The concern here is regulatory consistency rather than any need to keep the public constantly and precisely informed about the decisions being made and thus in a position to express itself.

In addition to these considerations involving procedural ethics (although in law, as in moral philosophy, the procedures represent the substance), the focal point of the discussion is the "ontological status" of the embryo, its primary definition. On this issue I believe that (for the time being) neither science nor philosophy nor theology can provide a universal, definitive, and acceptable interpretation. Moreover, I am convinced that the discussion of the "status of the embryo" is often tainted by overlapping interests, practical stresses and strains, and questions of principle. I am afraid, for example, that the insistence on the recognition of the embryo as a person, as well as the need to oppose those who consider it exclusively as a cluster of cells, is influenced by the attempt to modify the abortion laws and, ultimately, to have abortion classified as murder. Also, as in other domains linked to scientific research, there may be an overlap of principles and interests. For example, it seems obvious to me that the distinction proposed in the United

Kingdom by the Warnock Commission between *pre-embryo* (until the 14th day after fertilization) and a true embryo (after day 14) was strongly influenced by the pressing demand to find an ethical justification for experimentation on embryos. There is a strong analogy, now expressed in metascientific terms, between this distinction and the attempt of mediaeval theologians to make a chronological distinction between the embryo with a soul and the embryo without a soul, which God was supposed to infuse in the embryo only after the body had been prepared to receive it (the phenomenon described as *retarded animation*). Some theologians calculated that this literal incarnation of the soul took place 40 days after fertilization for males, 70 days after for females. Dante pushed this date even further forward, describing when the soul reaches the body: "si tosto come al feto / l'articular del cerebro è perfetto" (as soon as in the fetus / the articulation of the brain is perfect). This is a singular analogy between a mediaeval conception and the idea of Jacques Monod, according to which a person exists only when a complete electroencephalogram can be recorded.

Moreover, even present-day Catholic Church doctrine does not claim that every embryo is a person from the time of fertilization, but rather that it "could be": it is on the basis of this possibility that the Church demands a moral and legal protection equal to that for the child who has already been born. The thesis that "the embryo is one of us," which underlies the controversial document of the National Bioethics Committee, *Identity and Statute of the Human Embryo* (36), on the other hand, expresses a certainty. The argument that each of us was once an embryo, used to support this thesis, could be pushed much further: our species was indeed originally a sea animal, an amoeba, and even a molecule; each of us has been half ovum and half spermatozoon; each form of actual or potential life could thus be considered a moral subject and thus eligible for rigorous protection. What could lead to more peaceful discussions and responsible decisions is not, I believe, the dogma embryo = person but rather the assumption that the embryo contains the germ of a unique and unrepeatable individual (until its ultimate genetic duplication, whether spontaneous or induced). It is possible to reject this approach and even to claim that "the embryo is not a person" (37), although one cannot deny that it represents at least a project for human life and will become a man or a woman unless its development is interrupted by disease or some specific action. It is on this basis that the human embryo merits respect and protection; and the tendency is now towards recognition that no more embryos than are needed for medically assisted procreation should be produced, and their sale must be prohibited and experimentation on them restricted.

EMERGING PROBLEMS: HUMAN CLONING

To the three possible ways of having a child (natural procreation, medically assisted procreation, and adoption) has now been added a fourth, as announced in *Nature* on February 27, 1997: cloning. Cloning is the creation of a population of two or more individuals from a single stock, individuals thus genetically identical, and is familiar in both its natural and its artificially induced forms, the latter already produced by scientists for quite some time. Natural examples include the development of unfertilized eggs in insects and twin division in embryos. The sensation justly caused by the birth of the Scottish sheep Dolly stems from the technique used (use of somatic cells rather than germ cells), the fact that a mammal was involved, and, above all, the demonstration that it is therefore possible to artificially create human beings that are genetically identical to each other.

Identical? Not at all. There is no reason to be concerned: cloned individuals will grow up different from one another, because what is important in the formation of an individual is above all environment and education—not the genes. This is what was said by geneticists, starting from "the day after Dolly," in order to calm the alarmed moral reaction that immediately and spontaneously arose almost everywhere. Until February 26, 1997, it may be said (somewhat spitefully), many geneticists bent over backwards to demonstrate that all human qualities and perversities were due to the genes, repeating, confirming, or at least tolerating announcements of the discovery of genes that determined intelligence and stupidity, homosexuality, memory, aggressiveness and docility, delinquency, egoism and altruism, longevity, practically all diseases, virtue and vice, and all other human behavior.

By balancing out these opposite statements, some agreement may finally be reached to the effect that each individual is the result of multiple interrelated influences of the genes and the environment, with a variable prevalence of each factor according to the subject and the characteristics. Upstream from this observation, in any case, the technical feasibility and the will (deplored by some and encouraged by others) to clone human beings raises two moral questions. Is it right to proceed in this direction? Should the process be allowed or banned?

Before expressing an opinion on these issues, I need to make two distinctions. The first is necessitated by the fact that Italy's minister for health, shortly after the birth of Dolly, issued a decree banning all types of cloning, including that of animals. In this case, however, the bioethical problems are different: they refer to possible suffering, the issue of biodiversity, and other topics of "animal ethics." The second distinction is between *human beings* and *human cells and tissues*. Cells are already being cloned, and layers of human skin are produced (instead of skin removed from other parts of the body) for the treatment of burn patients. Any further expansion of such production (even of stem cells) for similar uses, or the development of cell or tissue cultures for the construction of organs or parts of organs for the purpose of transplants, should not in itself arouse any insurmountable moral controversy. Some controversy may of course arise over the origin, the use, and the distribution of such "materials."

Objections to the cloning of human beings are more substantial. In this case, analogical legitimation, according to which it is legitimate to create in the laboratory everything that nature produces spontaneously, is not valid. Hans Jonas wrote that cloning represents "the most despotic as regards method and in its purpose the most enslaving form of genetic manipulation; its aim is not an arbitrary modification of the hereditary substance but its equally arbitrary *fixation,* which is in contrast with the dominant strategy of nature" (38, p. 136).

In an attempt to account for the almost universal aversion for this technology (an aversion that has never occurred to the same extent and so rapidly for any other scientific discovery), one explanation pointed to our irrational fear that humans will end up usurping the role of the Creator. The more concrete objections are, however, of a completely different nature. Before discussing them, it is worth mentioning at least two reservations among the many raised, reservations that may seem tangential. There is concern over the potential for biological damage caused by the procedure—a concern reinforced by the 236 failures preceding the birth of Dolly, the problems seen in her subsequent growth, and the disproportion between the length of time required to evaluate the consequences and the hectic pace of modern-day research. Given time, however, any biological damage could be studied, reduced, and even eliminated. A second cause for concern is the horrible image of the creation of beings that are all the same. Owing to the multiple influences we are familiar with, this end could be pursued only by forcing the cloned beings to live in a highly uniform and totalizing environment, and even then it would not be possible to achieve. As the French Comité d'éthique wrote in its documented opinion on cloning: "The idea that a perfect genetic similarity in itself brings with it a perfect physical similarity totally lacks any scientific foundation" (see 39).

Paraphrasing Kant, the French committee developed a more substantial criticism: that all the proposed aims of cloning "share the feature of their principle consisting in planning the birth of one or more human beings not as a free end but as a pure means . . . which necessarily implies the exploitation of the person to be born." A reference to Kant is contained also in the opinion expressed, at the request of President Clinton, by the U.S. National Bioethics Advisory Committee: reproductive cloning means "treating persons as things," violating autonomy and personal freedom (40).

"Treating persons as things" describes succinctly the aim of possible cloners and their customers. Nearly 30 years ago Leon Kass drew up a list of cases proposed as favorable to cloning, defining it ironically as the "laundry list of possible applications, gradually becoming longer as we wait for the technique to be perfected" (41, cited in 38, p. 141). Now that cloning techniques, although still not perfect, are being applied, some items have been removed from Kass's list, possibly including certain projects whose motivation was once defined as "the need to beat the Russians and Chinese in this field," while others have been added, though many of these are open to criticism. One example is the possible cloning of individuals who are resistant to nuclear radiation or to other pollutants with the intention of using them in industrial processes or decontamination actions: there would be no damage to them and, arguably, many benefits for others. The obvious ethical drawback is that they would be created with a specific, limited function in mind; far from functioning as autonomous individuals, their destinies would not be their own to decide. Another example, one also supported on humanitarian grounds, is the possibility of enabling grieving parents to replace a beloved child killed in an accident with a duplicate obtained by cloning the dead child's cells. The new child would thus be conceived as the ghost of the dear one. Such a case could be seen as a manifestation of the freedom to procreate, but, in the case of conflict, I consider that the right to be born without predetermination is stronger.

In order to justify this and similar cases—in the argument that "if nature does it, why can't science?—proponents of cloning technology replace the word "nature" with the word "society." There is no doubt that society predetermines human fates—and how! So are we thus authorized to do so using technology? The preliminary question is, however, whether it is right for others to fix an individual's destiny from birth, in whatever direction, thus abolishing or at least tampering with her freedom of choice. It is true that this is done by nature, in the lottery that assigns different characteristics to different individuals, but the action of chance, which has neither will nor intention, does not give rise to any moral dilemmas. It is also true that society, a human creation, can fix an individual's destiny, since the location in which children are born and the different contexts of their growing up predetermine their futures to a greater or lesser degree. However, the history of human society, in its morally ascending line (which is not the only one) consists above all of attempting to modify the context in such a way that each individual can more freely decide her own destiny. If, on the other hand, society decided instead to add to the existing natural and societal limitations other predeterminations, sanctioned by science, in order to assemble a production line of customized human beings, this decision would not only violate the principle of personal rights. It would also make more difficult the other, less immediately profitable forms of genetic research that have already produced many results. And it would also reinforce "the conviction that the value of men and women does not depend on their personal identity but only on their biological qualities, qualities that may be coveted and thus selected" (42).

The innumerable variants in both the reasons for and the techniques of cloning will nevertheless ensure that an open and complex discussion continues on the first question I raised—whether it is right to proceed in this direction. And a possible answer to the second question of whether the process should be banned or allowed has in practice been given in the first "Additional Protocol" to the European Bioethical Convention, signed in Paris on January 11, 1998 (43). Article 1 states that "any intervention seeking to create a human being genetically identical to another human being, whether living or dead, is prohibited." The explanatory report accompanying the text condemns deliberate cloning as "a threat to human identity" and adds: "As naturally occurring genetic recombination is likely to create more freedom for a human being than a predetermined genetic makeup, it is in the interest of all persons to preserve the essentially random nature of the composition of their own genes."

There are other cases in which appeals have been made to the protection of law in the form of international legislation, to limit not scientific research but its methods and applications—as in, for instance, experiments on nonconsenting human beings or the manufacture or use of certain weapons (first chemical and bacteriological weapons, then nuclear weapons, and, more recently, antimen mines). Genetic predetermination of an individual, irrespective of whether it accounts for 1 or 90 percent of his ontogenesis (being determined also by environment, education, and personal choices), represents violence perpetrated on the unborn subject, resulting from a desire to impose on him the partial or total fate of a slave. The fact that this "other" subject has yet to be created does not change the substance of the argument.

Because cloning concerns both individuals and the human species, and because bans applying only in individual states would be ineffective, the correct approach is to aim at the approval and application of universal norms. That this approach is not without potential adherents is clear, both in view of the precedents mentioned above and also because the Council of Europe and the United States and other countries, as well as UNESCO and the World Health Organization, have already expressed concordant opinions on the subject. The ultimate goal is to have widely shared moral norms and universal legal norms.

REFERENCES

1. Shorter, E. *Storia del corpo femminile.* Feltrinelli, Milan, 1984 (*A History of Women's Bodies,* Basic Books, New York, 1982).
2. Mill, J. S. L'asservimento delle donne. In *La libertà.* RCS, Milan, 1999.
3. Encyclical, *Humanae vitae,* July 25, 1968, point 14: Vie illecite per la regolazione della natalità. Ed. Paoline, Milan, 1968.
4. Chiavacci, E., and Livi Bacci, M. *Etica e riproduzione: Un teologo e un demografo a confronto.* Le Lettere, Florence, 1995.
5. Kevles, D. J. Eugenics: Historical aspects. In *Encyclopedia of Bioethics,* edited by W. T. Reich, vol. 2, p. 766. Simon & Schuster, New York, 1995.
6. Kranz, H. W. *Die Gemeinshacftsunfahigen.* Giessen, 1939.
7. Ricciardi von Platten, A. *Il nazismo e l'eutanasia dei malati di mente,* p. 2. Le Lettere, Florence, 2000.
8. National Bioethies Committee. *Il problema bioetico della sterilizzazione non volontaria.* Rome, November 20, 1998.
9. Larkin, M. Male reproductive health: A hotbed of research. *Lancet* 352(9127): 552, 1998.
10. Vegetti Finzi, S. *Volere un figlio: La nuova maternità* fra natura e scienza. Mondadori, Milan, 1997.
11. Navarro, V. La politica alla guida dello stato sociale. *Qualità Equità* 14: 7–49, April-June 1998.

12. Golini, A. Le tendenze demografiche dell'Italia in un quadro europeo. In *Tendenze demografiche e politiche per la popolazione: Terzo rapporto IRP*, edited by A. Golini, p. 69. Il Mulino, Bologna, 1994.
13. National Bioethics Committee. Disuguaglianze. In *Infanzia e ambiente*, pp. 95–104. Poligrafico dello Stato, Rome, 1997.
14. United Nations Development Program. *Rapporto 1999 sullo sviluppo umano, 10: la globalizzazione.* Rosenberg & Sellier, Turin, 1999.
15. Sen, A. Missing women: Social inequality outweighs women's survival advantage in Asia and North Africa. *BMJ* 304: 587–588, 1992.
16. Furcht, A. *Alcuni contributi della demografia all'indagine biologica e alla riflessione etica,* pp. 6–7. Study Days on Population, Rome, January 7–9, 1997.
17. Monod, J. *Il caso e la necessità,* pp. 131–132. EST Mondadori, Milan, 1970.
18. Ruse, M. *Sociobiology: Sense or Nonsense?* Reidel, Dordrecht, 1979.
19. Steele, E. K., Lewis, S. E. M., and McClure, N. Science versus clinical adventurism in the treatment of azoospermia. *Lancet* 353: 516–517, 1999.
20. Tonini, E. Sulla fecondazione, l'Inghilterra di Blair inverte la rotta. *Avvenire,* July 28, 1999.
21. Engelhardt, H. T., Jr. *Manuale di bioetica.* Il Saggiatore, Milan, 1991.
22. Kant, I. *Fondazione della metafisica dei costumi,* p. 33. Laterza, Bari, 1997.
23. Hare, R. M. *Il pensiero morale.* Il Mulino, Bologna, 1989.
24. Jonas, H. *Il principio responsabilità: Un'etica per la civiltà tecnologica,* pp. 49–50. Einaudi, Turin, 1990.
25. National Bioethics Committee. *Parere sulle tecniche di procreazione assistita: Sintesi e conclusioni,* p. 12. Poligrafico dello Stato, Rome, 1995.
26. Cremona Law Courts, February 17, 1994. *Giurisprudenza italiana* 1(2): 996, 1994 (with a note by G. Ferrando).
27. Lanfranchi, V., and Favi, S. (eds.). *Figli della scienza: La riproduzione artificiale umana,* pp. 66–69. Editori Riuniti, Rome, 1988.
28. Kimbrell, A. *The Human Body Shop: The Engineering and Marketing of Life,* pp. 68–131. Harper Collins, London, 1993.
29. Berlinguer, G., and Garrafa, V. *La merce finale: Saggio sulla compravendita di parti del corpo umano,* pp. 60-69. Baldini and Castoldi, Milan, 1996.
30. Mancia, M. Vita prenatale e organizzazione della mente. In *La nascita del sé,* edited by M. Ammanniti. Laterza, Rome, 1989.
31. Vegetti Finzi, S. Famiglia e identità femminile nell'epoca della tecnica. In *Famiglia 'generativa' o famiglia 'riproduttiva?* edited by E. Scabini and G. Rossi, p. 195. Vita e pensiero, Milan, 1999.
32. Harvard Divinity School and J. P. Kennedy Jr. Foundation. *Abortion, a Dilemma of Our Time* (based on the proceedings of the 1st International Congress on Abortion, Washington, D.C., 1967). Etas Kompass, Milan, 1970.
33. Berlinguer, G. *La legge sull'aborto.* Editori Riuniti, Rome, 1978.
34. Encyclical of John Paul II, *Evangelium vitae,* March 25, 1995, points 58-59: Il valore e l'inviolabilità della vita umana. Ed. Paoline, Milan, 1995.
35. *Convenzione per la protezione dei diritti dell'uomo e della dignità dell'essere umano in rapporto alla biomedicina.* Oviedo, April 4, 1997. (Also known as *Convenzione bioetica europea* or *Convenzione di Oviedo.*)

36. National Bioethics Committee. *Identità e statuto dell'embrione umano,* June 22, 1996. Poligrafico dello Stato, Rome, 1997.
37. Mori, M. *Aborto e morale.* Il Saggiatore-Flammarion, Milan, 1996.
38. Jonas, H. *Tecnica medicina ed etica: Prassi del principio responsabilità.* Einaudi, Turin, 1997.
39. *Les Cahiers du Comité consultatif national d'éthique pour les sciences de la vie et de la santé,* Vol. 12, pp. 17–39. Paris, July 1997.
40. National Bioethics Advisory Committee. Document f. 31b–32b. June 1997.
41. Kass, L. R. New beginning in life. In *The New Genetics and the Future of Man,* edited by M. P. Hamilton, pp. 43–63. Grand Rapids, Michigan, 1972.
42. Pontificia Accademia Pro Vita. Riflessioni sulla clonazione. *L'Osservatore Romano,* June 25, 1997, p. 7.
43. *Additional Protocol to the Convention on Human Rights and Dignity of the Human Being with Regard to the Application of Biology and Medicine, on the Prohibition of Cloning Human Beings.* Council of Europe, DIR/JUR (97), 14.

CHAPTER 2

Population, Ethics, and Equity

INDIVIDUAL CHOICES AND COLLECTIVE DECISIONS

As population dynamics and the individual and collective decisions affecting it are gradually subjected not only to analysis and statistical forecasting, but also to moral judgment, growing differences of interpretation and the need for further scrutiny emerge. On the one hand, conflicting interpretations make efforts to define policies and goals in public affairs, based on the idea of fundamental ethical norms, far more difficult. Such efforts, of course, find an important and demanding area of implementation in demographic problems. Many problems demanding ethical evaluation have emerged with striking clarity in recent years, such as the government of migration, the relations between men and women and between generations, and the relationship among population, environment, and resources. On the other hand, these differences involve individual choices in which the principles of autonomy and responsibility are intertwined, especially in the areas of genetics, healing, sexuality and procreation (natural and assisted), and the problems of the terminal stages of life—all aspects of human existence that are increasingly affected by advances in the biomedical sciences.

I ran into some difficulties as I attempted to wend my way through the ethical issues related to these matters. The first difficulty was the scope of the problems, as illustrated by the above examples. I sought a brief outline for reference purposes in the new edition of the *Encyclopedia of Bioethics,* edited by W. T. Reich (1). There I found an extensive entry on Population Ethics that contained a number of subheadings: "Normative Approaches," "Religious Traditions," "Population Policies," "Fertility Control Strategies," "Migrations and Refugees." To this must be added, from other parts of the five-volume encyclopedia, many more related topics: Death and Dying, Eugenics, Aging and the Aged, Euthanasia and Sustaining Life, Freedom and Coercion, Epidemics, Sexuality, Children, Future Generations (Obligations to), Reproductive Technologies, Food Policy, Race and Racism, Women, International Health, Environmental Policy and Law, Abortion, Genetics and Environment in Human Health, and Marriage and Other Domestic Partnerships. I was unsure whether to interpret the length of this still incomplete list of topics as a sign of the invasive tendency of bioethics or as a demonstration of the moral force of population-related issues. In any case, I found in it a confirmation of the interrelatedness of the issues emerging at the cutting edge of science with issues central to everyday experience, today and yesterday.

The second difficulty was procedural, not substantive. It arose when I went on to examine the language of science as used in studies of population demography. As I proceeded, I gradually realized that in this science, perhaps more than in others, many words are imbued not only with a descriptive meaning but also with an implied positive or negative value—that is, with moral attributes. In other words, the objectivity of the statistics is thus intertwined with the subjectivity of its conceptual categories.

WORDS AND VALUES IN DEMOGRAPHY

The words used in demography and their meanings obviously change over time and according to scientific progress. The present-day classification of the causes of death, for example, has very little in common with the list drawn up by John Graunt in London in 1632 or with the nomenclature proposed by William Farr in the years 1839–1840, which, in a way appropriate to the knowledge available and to the state of society prevailing at the time, divided the causes of death into three fundamental groups: epidemic, sporadic, and violent.

However, words and meanings also change according to the ideology and moral criteria of those who introduce and use them, as can be seen in many examples. Although the first declaration of rights and all subsequent declarations have proclaimed that "all men are created equal," demography long made a distinction between legitimate children and those deemed illegitimate because they were born out of wedlock. The distinction was long used not just for the purpose of statistical classification but also to stigmatize. In Papal Rome, a further category was devised for the children of unknown mothers who, unable or unwilling to keep them, in the dead of night used to push their newborns through a revolving window known as the *ruota* at hospitals and convents. Each foundling was lovingly cared for, but was branded as *figlio di m. ignota*, "child of an unknown m. [mother]." Tradition has it that deleting the period in the Italian expression and doubling the "t" gave rise to one of the worst insults in Roman dialect ("son of a mignotta!"), although learned etymologists consider that the swear word comes from the French *mignote*, "favorite," itself derived from *mignonne*, "pretty one."

In actual fact, the distinction made between legitimate and illegitimate children must be attributed to customs and laws that either acknowledged or prescribed such a distinction rather than to demographers. It continued to be used in Italy until an act passed on October 31, 1955, established that all public deeds and documents should contain details pertaining only to the subjects and not to their parents. Subsequently, the term "illegitimate" fell into disuse in demography as well. Slightly earlier, the same thing happened to another term, *stirpe*, used to refer to persons or peoples of high lineage or superior descent, widely used in the language of the fascist period to claim the superiority of ancient Romans (and therefore of modern Italians) over any other people. The word survived the fall of fascism, appearing in title X of the Penal Code (known as the Rocco Code, after the minister of justice at the time), promulgated in the 1930s, which lumped together as *Delitti contro la integrità e la sanità della stirpe* (Offenses against the integrity and health of the race) numerous acts related to sexuality and reproduction: abortion, induced inability to procreate, encouragement of practices against procreation, and infection with syphilis and gonorrhea. These were considered serious offenses because they ran counter to the state's demographic interest.

The same code defined sexual violence in anatomical terms as *violenza carnale* (rape). Rape was notably included in penal law, and thus in court statistics, as one of the offenses *contro la moralità pubblica e il buon costume* (against morality), not among those against the individual (e.g., murder, bodily harm, assault, and battery). Only 40 years after the fall of fascism was the offense placed in its correct context, in the face of bitter resistance from many Catholics, with the acknowledgment that the primary harm is caused to the woman as a person. Moreover, not only actual penetration but any other form of sexual act under duress was then acknowledged as a violent act within the purview of the law.

A further example is the word "homosexuality," in itself morally neutral. As is well known, however, the practice has often been associated with guilt and is still proscribed in the penal codes of a number of countries. What is less well known is that, in international medical nomenclature, it has been considered a pathological entity on a par with other diseases. This remained the case until scientific progress and civil rights movements abolished the connection, at least in disease statistics. But stigmata come and go. In everyday language, and here and there in statistical surveys of the E.U. countries, the word *extracomunitario* ("coming from outside the E.U.") is used to define many immigrants (though, of course, not those from Japan, Canada, or the United States). The persons in question are classified on the basis of their non-membership in a geopolitical community, although the boundary thus created tends to exclude them also from the community of living persons. The term is spreading and is now used also by many of those working to ensure the reception of these individuals.

In other cases, we could speak of words that are omitted rather than uttered. One of these is "hunger," which is ignored in mortality statistics even though hunger is still directly or indirectly (owing to its associated diseases and diminished immune defenses) one of the main causes of death throughout the world. It should be noted that it was explicitly *included* in the early documents of modern demographic science. In the "Natural and Political Observations upon the Bills of Mortality" (presented by John Graunt to the Royal Society; 2), six persons were reported as having been found dead of starvation in the streets of London in 1632. Another term related to premature death, "poverty," was used only in 1955, after a long silence on the subject on the part of the World Health Organization, by the WHO director general. While presenting the report, *The State of World Health,* he stated that poverty is "the main cause of death in the world" (3).

However, the word itself has never appeared in those mortality statistics classified by cause of death. One could argue that the direct clinical cause of death is always something else, never poverty itself, but this could also indicate medicine's tendency (to a greater extent than in demographic science) to "medicalize" every aspect of human life, using aseptic terms that disguise differences and conflicts in social relations.

This tendency could also account for the epidemiological transition, that is, the shift from infectious diseases, caused by viruses, microorganisms, and parasites, to chronic-degenerative (or, more accurately, noninfectious) diseases, such as cancer and cardiovascular, neural, mental, endocrine, and stress-related disorders, as predominant causes of illness and death. "The decline of the first pathology," wrote Giulio A. Maccararo, "announced the gradual clearing of natural causes of disease from the environment; the onset of the second betrays the corruption of the same environment by artificial causes of disease" (4). Or, interpreted in a more illuminating fashion, this change in the description of disease actually represents a "passage from a pathology of man as an animal, a pathology widely shared with or even transmitted by other species, to a pathology of man as such, and indeed highly anthropogenic in both its specificity and origin."

It is easy to see the moral implications involved in either neglecting the facts or concealing them behind a useful but purely descriptive analysis of the epidemiological transition: first, that the past was dominated by physiogenic diseases due mainly to natural causes (including infections, nutritional deficiencies, and climate), with humans as passive objects or secondary agents with respect to disease factors present in the external environment; and second, that most diseases are now anthropogenic, due mainly, although not exclusively, to changes brought about through human action or inaction. As a corollary to this observation, I could add that hospital infections caused by negligence or by germs that have become resistant through the abuse of drugs, although representing a dramatically widespread phenomenon, are either ignored or only reluctantly included in disease statistics. It is significant that, under another name and other clinical conditions, often fatal at the time, hospital infections were for a long time classified as gangraena nosocomialis, until the acceptance in 1898 of the proposal of the demographer J. Bertillon that they should be included (and concealed) in the group of "purulent infections and septicemias." The current silence on this topic in official statistics, despite the published research on the subject (reports read only by specialists, however), shows that the resistance and hostility encountered by Semmelweiss in Vienna in 1847, when he clearly demonstrated that the high mortality due to puerperal sepsis was caused by infections transmitted to women by the hands of physicians and students during childbirth (for which demonstration he was subjected to persecution), are not just a remote black chapter in the history of medicine.

Lastly, I should like to point out the scientific incorrectness and consequent ethical implications of two other definitions commonly used in statistics. One is the concept of spontaneous abortion. As the word "spontaneous" here refers to what happens in the absence of human intervention, abortion may be said to be spontaneous only when natural factors are the cause, factors such as the mother's age and parity, incurable pathologies during pregnancy, or selective factors in the embryo—factors, in any event, not dependent on avoidable risks. In many cases, however, abortion caused unintentionally but the result of harmful action is also classified as spontaneous, such as that due to accident or violence, to environmental or workplace factors, to preventable disease, or to conditions of stress in the pregnant woman. Also, genetic alterations in the gametes that can produce an anomalous embryo doomed to abortion may not always be in the category of "spontaneous." They are frequently caused by harmful factors, such as radiation and toxic substances, to which one or both parents are exposed in the workplace (5).

Because the word "spontaneous" suggests the ineluctability of the phenomenon and may thus lead to resignation, the extensive and improper (because potentially absolving) use of the term "spontaneous abortion" can be the cause of clear-cut conceptual and practical omissions. To which may be added, again on the subject of abortion, a short comment on another commonly used expression that also implies a value judgment and is almost always incorrect: "therapeutic abortion." This definition is correct only in cases of interruptions of pregnancy for the purpose of treating a serious ongoing disease in the mother or to prevent risk to her life, situations now rare, given current medical progress. However, this expression is normally used to refer to abortions practiced in cases of fetal anomalies revealed by the increasingly widespread application of prenatal diagnostic techniques: a strange "therapy" in this case, as it brings to an end the very life that it claims to benefit. The incorrectness of the term merely conceals the fact that this practice is actually a selective abortion: a practice that, unlike truly spontaneous abortions, gives rise to complex moral reflection (6).

The other definition to be examined involves the distinction made between endogenous mortality and exogenous mortality. I have dwelt at greater length on this topic elsewhere (7) and limit myself here to a few observations. Obviously, many deaths are due to typical endogenous (e.g., genetic) causes and others to typical exogenous (e.g., violent) causes. The relationship between the two, however, has been subject to many different interpretations over time. The late nineteenth century was characterized, in the wake of discoveries in microbiology, by the idea that external enemies (microorganisms) were the cause of all disease. The late twentieth century was apparently committed to finding a single defect—today a gene—responsible for each nosological condition (as well as, in the worst positivist anthropological tradition, for all human behavior deemed abnormal). Also, the conceptions of "exogenous" and "endogenous" have been modified several times in the light of cultural factors (such as scientific discoveries) and of changes in the objective description of diseases. An example of this is the change in knowledge and theories about the origin and evolution of tumors.

The main point here is that diseases often represent the body's focal point in the relationship between internal and external environments, that is, between individual predisposition and personal behavior on the one hand and hazardous living and working conditions on the other. To lay the blame exclusively on the outside, that is, on nature (germs or other external factors), or exclusively on the inside, that is, on the individual (the genes), can lead to epistemological blindness concerning the complexity and diversity of disease-causing factors. Alternatively, such misguided fault-finding can paralyze efforts to ward off attack from germs and other factors present in the environment (which mainly affect weaker subjects) or to avoid a proneness to disease becoming actual disease or leading to death (on this topic, see 8). Any of these tendencies can stand in the way of proposals for adequate governmental and other measures aimed at preventive health care, proposals which, as William Farr (9) wrote, "represent one of the goals of mortality statistics."

THE ETHICAL BASES OF POPULATION
POLICIES

According to Donald W. Warwick, population ethics is supported by two pillars—moral principles and factual information (10). He stresses the importance of knowing and telling the truth, which means providing "accurate information about population policies and avoiding lies, misrepresentations, and evasions about their content, implementation, and consequences." Because the truth is related not only to the data themselves but also to the way in which they are collected, classified, and interpreted, I thought it would be a good idea to begin from a criticism of the "misrepresentations, distortions, and omissions" arising from a scientifically unsuitable and morally tendentious use of certain words. I cannot guarantee that the choice of these examples and my comments are not likewise flawed by a particular experience and point of view. However, I am convinced of the validity of the critical exercise of reflecting on these and other words (past and present) used in demography, as their use almost always carries a moral meaning that it is only honest to bring to the surface.

Farr's comment quoted above (9) could serve as a guide for the following discussion. It is based on the notion that practical or moral philosophy (ethics) involves choosing what is right and distinguishing between good and bad, which further entails inquiring as to the relationship between ethics and the governing of public issues—which includes, or should include (because of their intrinsic importance and growing significance), policies designed to deliberately modify the population in its number and structure.

At the outset, the principal ethical question is whether it is fitting for the institutions in this field to pursue "purposeful aims" and to decide on "action aimed to interfere deliberately with reality" (11), that is, by means of decisions affecting the sphere of personal freedom. Nevertheless, it may be claimed that all policies—not only demographic policies but also those concerning the economy, the environment, health, social status, territory, international relations, and so forth—have an effect on the population. While maintaining the importance of personal freedom, the moral discourse thus shifts towards the motivation, purpose, and form of the choices.

These arguments are not easy to debate, especially in Italy and Germany, where, more than 50 years after the fall of fascism and Nazism, a certain hostility is still displayed towards any conscious demographic policy. The suspicion is that any action in this field will almost inexorably lead back to the aberrations of fascism, which sought military power by increasing the number of soldiers (the dream was to deploy "eight million bayonets"), or of Nazism, which carried out sterilization of the weak, compulsory eugenics, and genocide. Similar phenomena, although in different forms and with different impacts, still occur today, as in, for instance, the ethnic cleansing carried out in southeastern Europe and other parts of the world.

On the other hand, what can replace conscious choice? Very often, prejudice. One typical example is the attitude towards immigration. It can hardly be denied that, in today's world, even though one may hope from a moral standpoint that, one day, frontiers will no longer exist and unrestricted travel will be possible anywhere in the world, setting rules and limits to the movement of populations is still expedient and perhaps even right. This, indeed, was the claim made by Immanuel Kant in his philosophical project "Per la pace perpetua" (For a Perpetual Peace) (12):

> It is not philanthropy, but law, and therefore hospitality means the right of a foreigner not be treated with hostility when he lands on the soil of someone else. The latter can send away the former when this can be done without his ruin; but as long as the foreigner remains peacefully in his place, he may not be greeted with hostility. It is not a right to hospitality which gives rise to this claim (for this purpose a special contract of benevolence would be required, in order to make the foreigner a co-inhabitant for a certain period of time) but a right to visit, which all men are entitled to, to propose themselves as members of the society on the grounds of a right to the common possession of the surface of the earth. In this way distant continents can entertain peaceful mutual relations that later become regulated by laws, and can thus ultimately lead mankind increasingly closer to a cosmopolitan constitution.

What is less right, and may even have serious consequences, is to consider immigration as an impending disaster and the root of all evils, or to introduce rules determining, on the strength of alleged qualitative criteria, which human beings are and which are not to be allowed to cross a frontier.

The concept of superior and inferior human races, developed historically during the nineteenth century (13), was extensively used to codify such discriminatory rules, especially in Europe and the United States. However, it is only right to acknowledge that the most fruitful example of immigration and the mingling of human races in modern times is the foundation and development of the United States of America. The positive outcome of this event is overshadowed by the numerous trials endured over time by Native Americans, African Americans, and other ethnic groups, by the persistence of discrimination, and by measures introduced in various periods to set immigrant quotas according to each group's racial affinity with Anglo-Saxon stock (14). In many respects, however, the development of the United States has an exemplary history.

Nevertheless, its positive aspects have not been sufficiently appreciated and assimilated in Europe. Many European countries (including Italy) were, in the short span of a few decades, transformed from countries of emigrants into countries with a strong immigrant influx. This has raised concern in Italy that the incoming tide of foreigners will leave young people jobless, bring diseases, and so corrupt the Italian species that (according to the forecasts of certain population experts), if the birth rate remains low, the population of Italian origin will disappear completely in 150 to 200 years. On this last subject I should like to make a personal comment. I was born on the isolated island of Sardinia, and I have a secret hope that, in some mountain village of this land, a few specimens of *Homo sardus* will survive, at least until the year 2200. According to studies by Cavalli Sforza (15), this population, like the Basques, is genetically distinct from the Mediterranean peoples who have profoundly and fruitfully mingled. Regarding the other reasons for concern, it should be pointed out that immigrants do not steal jobs but do work that Italians no longer want to do. And, with a few rare exceptions, they do not bring diseases but rather contract them after their arrival in Italy; they are actually among the healthiest citizens of their native countries and, thus, the fittest for immigration (16).

When there is no actual prejudice, population policies are occasionally replaced by rhetoric. A typical example is that of the family, a topic linked to procreation and to relations between generations. I know of no other country in Europe in which treacly family rhetoric is so blatantly accompanied by an almost total lack of material support for married couples and children. Public policy in Italy "has completely neglected the family and has actually penalized it to a considerable extent in legislation on housing, employment, taxation, and family allowances" (17). Analyses show that social expenditure in Italy is roughly at the same level as in the European Union as a whole, but in Italy it is strongly tilted in favor of old-age and retirement pensions rather than payments to families and young people in the form of family allowances, job training, social services, and other welfare benefits. The problem of intergenerational inequity therefore tends to be aggravated.

Leaving aside the obstacles due to prejudice and rhetoric, what possible trends can be established in the relationship between ethics and population policies? Even where there are no codified rules, on the grounds that legislation that encroaches upon individual choices is not necessary and may even be dangerous, the fact remains that both individuals and institutions always base their decisions both on material considerations and on more or less explicitly stated moral values. Of course, a number of different options exist in this field, but a broad common awareness has arisen, which I shall adopt as my thesis here. It is rooted in the idea that the secular and democratic state must base its rules and decisions, not on religion or ideology, but on three fundamental principles: human rights, pluralism of ideas and behavior, and the pursuit of common goals. Of course, the relative importance of such goals changes according to the period, but equity remains central as both the purpose and the basis of human society.

THE ANTITHESIS: THE ETHICAL STATE

I shall come back to these three points—rights, pluralism, and equity—later. First, I need to present an opposite thesis that will serve to clarify the meaning of an idea that has arisen and that persists in a number of countries—both in dictatorships of all kinds and in nations in which religion has been adopted as the basis of social order. This is the idea of the "ethical state" that, insofar as it is based on an intrinsic ethic, incorporates individuals' demands, acknowledges only one morality as valid, and dictates norms for how citizens should behave. This idea has spanned the centuries and has almost always entailed constraints or suggestions (often accompanied by the promise of benefits or the threat of punishment). Examples abound throughout history; from Plato's eugenic ideas, in which it was in the interest of the state for the best men to mate with the best women in order to perfect the élite, to the demographic policies implemented by fascism and Nazism, down to the recent introduction in India and then in China of a birth control system including rewards, punishments, and coercive measures.

To some extent this idea of the ethical state pervades even the democratic nations (including Italy): for instance, in the area of procreation. Certain provisions of Italy's Rocco Penal Code, which meted out prison sentences to "whoever publicly incites or advertises practices against procreation," outlived the fall of fascism by several decades, until they were finally repealed by the Constitutional Court. This topic still arouses hostility and negative, sometimes threatening, reactions in the religious and political circles opposed to sex education (or information) in schools. Such hostility again appeared after the onset of the AIDS crisis, despite its serious possible consequences for young people's lives. The opponents of sex information initiated an assault on two fronts: the Education Ministry, which was told it must not interfere, as sex education is the responsibility of families, and the Health Ministry, which was told it must not recommend the use of condoms, as this might encourage immoral sexual conduct. The attempt was to stop the state from performing its duty of educating and of preventing disease. This is an omission that, morally, is as open to criticism as is enforcing an obligation to behave in a certain way.

A third variant in the methods used by the ethical state, in addition to constraint and omission, is interfering in individuals' choices by prohibiting and punishing.

One example in Italy is that of the first artificial insemination bills presented to parliament as soon as the techniques began to appear. The bills were peremptory in classifying these techniques as legal offenses, specifying jail sentences of up to three years for "a married woman who agrees to artificial heterologous insemination, even with the husband's consent," for "an unmarried woman who agrees to be artificially inseminated" (in this case, with any semen), for "married couples requesting and agreeing to homologous artificial insemination" (i.e., also including the husband), for "physicians who are accessories to the offense," and lastly for "anyone who practices artificial insemination in a woman, even with her consent" (18). We can identify two underlying ethical issues in this trend. One stems from the concept that only what is natural is good, while all that is artificial is evil and sinful and thus a criminal offense. The other consists of the fact that accepting a donor's semen, "even with the husband's consent" (as he is obviously suffering from some reproductive disorder), amounts to adultery and must be punished as such.

Significantly, the bill proposed in 1959 added that "the husband can refuse to recognize a child conceived in wedlock by heterologous insemination," even in a case in which the husband had given his consent—a provision that tallies with article 235 of the Civil Code, which provides for non-recognition of a child in cases of impotence, absence, separation, and adultery. Much emphasis is correctly laid on the fact that in procreation, whether natural or assisted, the most important subject from the ethical point of view is the child to be born. In the case cited here, a desired child would have been deprived of all protection.

Replacing the concept of the ethical state with that of a state based on individual freedom certainly does not mean doing away with the need for rules based, in one way or another, on moral principles. As must be acknowledged, however, principles and rules on procreating and giving birth, living and aging, falling ill and being healed, settling down and migrating, and dying—that is, individual events that in sum define the behavior of the whole population—are much more complicated. Nevertheless, if the rules are based on rights, pluralism, and freely chosen common aims, they are more heavily imbued with personal opportunities that are acknowledged and protected than is a mere translation of religious principles, or totalitarian ideologies, into constraining legislation.

I now return to the fundamental principles outlined earlier: human rights, pluralism, and equity.

HUMAN RIGHTS

In the area of human rights, we can go back to the solemn and universally valid declarations of principles made in the late eighteenth century in America and France, incorporated into the constitutions of many nations and updated in the twentieth century in the United Nations Declaration. The numerous instances of violations of these rights in 1999 stole the limelight during the celebration of the

50th anniversary of the U.N. document, violations that led observers to describe the Declaration as "a Charter betrayed." That description is too absolute in that it neglects the progress actually made, and too discouraging in that it reinforces the common claim that the Declaration "may be right in principle but not in practice." Immanuel Kant dwelt at length on this aphorism in 1793 (19). His argument was that the concept could be justified only "for empty ideas, which would find no use in practice or even be detrimental to it. But in a theory based on the concept of duty, any concern over the empty ideality of this concept disappears completely." The presumptuous and contemptuous tone used by those who would "reform reason through experience" is, according to Kant, an expression of "the conceited idea that it is possible to see further and more clearly with a mole's eyes rooted on experience rather than with eyes given to a being who was born to stand erect and admire the heavens."

When we look at the world, although it is difficult to strike a balance between the good and the evil found in it, we cannot deny that statements of rights have been responsible for much good and should, therefore, be implemented. Scientific knowledge and social change nevertheless call for a constant updating. I shall try to explain the moral and juridical implications of this need by means of several points made in a contemporary document that is consistent with the U.N. Declaration, namely, the Constitution of the Italian Republic, which came into effect on January 1, 1948, and which represents principles also subscribed to in many other European constitutions of that time.

The statement of these principles begins with three articles proclaiming the inviolability of personal freedom (art. 13), of one's household and freedom of residence (art. 14), and of the freedom and confidentiality of the mail and all other forms of correspondence (art. 15). The only exception is for action taken by the judicial authorities, and then only in cases and in ways provided for by law. But what has changed, particularly in the area of information and communication, since the Constitution came into effect?

On the one hand, a new right was established in fact and in law: citizens' right to be informed, even when ill, of all that pertains to their own health, and to be empowered to decide their own fate on the basis of a practical recognition of the ethical concept of personal autonomy. For example, the expression "informed consent," now accepted even by the Code of Medical Ethics, denotes a move away from the paternalistic idea of physicians alone having access to information and deciding on treatment. In addition to the elementary right to be treated, informed consent also implies having the right to request and obtain interruption of treatment and the right to refuse any therapy in the case of disagreement, even to the extent of being allowed to die. It has also been established that both workers in factories and residents in local communities have the right to be informed of risks deriving from potential sources of hazard in their environments. In recent years, this legislation has been the driving force behind openly conducted research in the field of environmental epidemiology for the purpose of disease prevention.

On the other hand, there has been an exponential increase in the collection and transmission of information, including even the most intimate data relating to our personal lives. This has come about not only as a result of the greater ease with which data can be gathered and processed, but also due to several coinciding factors: (*a*) advances in biomedicine, which, for instance, paved the way to genetic identity testing; (*b*) market and political pressures to ascertain and exploit citizens' habits as expressed in consumer patterns or through opinion polls; (*c*) the spread of demographic and social surveys; and, above all, (*d*) electronic data collection for the purpose of setting up public and private databases, both overt and covert, in which each of us, often without our knowledge, is classified in a dozen different ways. All this may have the positive effect of an improved knowledge of individuals and of the population as a whole. However, it is also liable to represent a greater danger to the individual's right to privacy than are the violations of the "household" and "confidentiality of correspondence" referred to in the Constitution (as well as in the Penal Code, in which these violations are labeled offenses). This may also have a negative effect on access to other rights. One of the most controversial areas is genetic screening, which has been used both to selectively regulate access to the workplace and to reduce the cost to the employer of health care covered by private insurance. European legislation seems to be oriented towards prohibiting the use of genetic tests for employment or insurance purposes that could be detrimental to individuals (20).

In the field of statistical surveys, also, demographers have encountered morally and legally complex situations, in relation, for instance, to the conduct of a census when there is a conflict between the need to obtain information about the population and moral doubts concerning the legitimacy of some of the questions. What is odd, however, is the far greater outcry over some apparently indiscreet questions than over the failure to ask other questions in no way embarrassing, questions indispensable for obtaining a complete picture of the population's characteristics. One such much-needed question is on social class, information that has been requested and processed by the U.K. Registrar General for over a century, while in Italy it has only recently been considered essential to an understanding of the country's demographic and social structure and the differences in health conditions. Sometimes a venial sin of commission is deemed more serious than a genuinely serious sin of omission.

Another increasingly controversial issue is alluded to in article 29, according to which "the Republic recognizes the rights of the family as a natural society based on marriage." Although the existence of couples formed on the basis of other criteria is not a new phenomenon, what is new is the increasing frequency of such partnerships and the attitude towards these couples: although classified as anomalous under article 29, they are treated as normal in everyday society. Many have also requested (and sometimes obtained) some formal recognition, and they are also increasingly taken into account in demographic interpretations. Moral evaluations of these nonstandard families hover between two opposite considerations: is the phenomenon disruptive, or is it an updated confirmation of the validity of the family as an institution? A practical question that is being asked increasingly often is, to what extent can the law defend and legitimate cases of families at some remove from "normalcy," such as homosexual couples or polygamous families within other religious and juridical traditions?

In the area of health, the Constitution's main statement is expressed in article 32: "The Republic safeguards health as a fundamental right of the individual and as a public interest." This wording not only has stood the test of time but has even anticipated events. Based on this principle and following the latest advances in medicine, a widespread demand emerged in Italy in the 1960s and 1970s, focused principally on disease prevention, which made health care available to all citizens. In its article 32, Italian legislation has recently acknowledged also the ethical stimulus and the legal justification for ensuring access to health services for immigrants, even illegal ones. This provision stems from recognition that, although not citizens, immigrants are individuals with the same needs as any others. The word "individual" is significantly used only in this article of the Constitution; in all others, reference is made to the "citizen." The word chosen represents also a tacit acknowledgment that it is in the community interest for non-citizens to be cared for, even if only to prevent the spread of disease.

As Paolo De Sandre writes, the consideration that rights are fundamental to collective and individual choices in the demographic field may also imply "the growing importance of public regulation of private affairs" (11, pp. 459–460). Public regulation can be a cause of private inconvenience and moral problems: "In many essential aspects of an individual's life (education, work, health, welfare) as it gradually unfolds, the interlocutor is in each case the institutional system, the functioning of which is governed by norms of public interest. The predominance of this relationship, which has in varying degrees replaced the existing inter-personal support networks, is such as to overshadow in their subjective perception the advantage that these networks of persons may deserve in the various stages of life, particularly when they are made up of persons belonging to successive generations." It could be added that, as Salvatore Veca has stressed, there is also a danger of diminishing the value of personal responsibility and commitment, as well as of aggravating the (to some extent physiological) tensions between the individual's right to well-being and to equity—rights that must be reconciled or, rather, allowed to coexist (21).

THE VALUE OF PLURALISM

The second fundamental principle is pluralism. Pluralism is a want to be redressed and it is merely a fact. This obviously does not imply that any personal choice is *ipso facto* morally legitimate. However, we must consider that reducing everything *ad unum* would (besides being unfair, as pluralism is an individual right and a resource for everyone) require coercive measures that are incompatible with today's democratic societies. In areas sensitive to rapid change, in particular as a result of technological progress or of behavioral models that have broken with tradition, two aims should be pursued: the creation of a widely shared and freely accepted "common awareness" that is respectful of personal choices and, at the same time, a system of rules capable both of settling the inevitable conflicts arising over values with as few prohibitions as possible and of bringing out the positive goals. Achieving these two aims is anything but easy under any conditions, and particularly when controversial issues tend to be forced onto ideologically irreconcilable grounds. Nevertheless, this appears to be the only possible path to follow. In Chapter 1, I referred to one of life's extreme events: birth. I shall now deal more concisely with the other extreme: death.

The free choice of whether, when, and how to procreate obviously is not reflected in any such freedom at the end of life, since (at the present time) death is a destiny shared by human beings and all other living creatures. However, there can be freedom of choice about not whether, but how and, within certain time constraints, when to die. The moral reflections on this issue have in the past revolved mainly around suicide. Giacomo Leopardi reflected on the subject (22, nn. 815–816, p. 194):

> I am fully aware that nature abhors suicide with all its might. I am aware that this violates all its laws more seriously than any other human sin; but since nature has been totally altered and our life has ceased to be natural, since the happiness destined to us by nature has vanished for ever and we have become irremediably unhappy because of that death wish that, according to nature, we should never even have conceived of; that, despite nature and through the force of reason, has indeed taken possession of us: why does reason itself prevent us from satisfying it and from remedying in the only possible way the damage that it alone has caused us?

For a long time, when religion had a more profound and widespread influence on human behavior, a ban was placed on suicide, because the body was conceived of as, in a real sense, sacred. In such circumstances, to reject suicide may have represented for an individual the "free choice" to accept and obey a doctrine. But it became anything but free when suicide was written into the statute books as a criminal offense, with punishment meted out: if the attempt proved unsuccessful, the would-be suicide was punished; if successful, his goods were confiscated in order to punish his heirs.

Moral reflections are now focused more on euthanasia than on suicide. These two issues—suicide and euthanasia—are of great intrinsic importance, and thinking about them will help us appreciate more fully human essence, values, and relational systems. Nevertheless, particularly in the discussion of euthanasia, I

2. Population, Ethics, and Equity / 45

should like to point out that anyone consulting the bioethics literature, or aware of the space devoted by the media to discussions on this topic, gets the impression that the world is full of people with nothing else on their minds but dying or having themselves helped to die as quickly as possible. Euthanasia is an issue of the greatest ethical import, of course. This would be true even if it concerned only a single person, because it is literally a matter of life and death. I have already mentioned that one of the decisions concerning one's own fate that must be included under personal autonomy is the choice of whether to continue being treated in the event of a serious illness. This desire can be expressed in the form of a "life testament" or "living will," a legal provision already adopted in several countries that allows individuals to indicate the decisions to be made about treatment (possibly by a named "trustee") should they no longer be in a position to voice such decisions. This solution is widely accepted and can be considered a free choice. However, the idea of allowing physicians to deliberately administer substances leading to death rightly encounters considerable resistance.

Nevertheless, in the vast majority of cases, what the "terminally ill" want is not active or passive euthanasia. What they really want is to be aided, to receive comfort and company, to have their pain soothed, and not to be subjected to useless and cruel therapies. In other words, their primary freedom is to be allowed to die with the least possible pain and the greatest possible dignity. I should like to add that the world is populated with people who want to live as long as possible; therefore, what is significant in the demographic, social, and moral fields is the widespread existence and persistence, despite all of the progress in medicine, of events that might be classified as "cacothanasia"—bad death—owing to both the way in which these events occur and their premature and untimely nature. This includes deaths that could have been avoided or delayed if suitable preventive measures had been taken or effective therapies promptly deployed.

Death in general may be appraised from the point of view that it "serves life," because "the natural order is a cycle of destruction, reproduction, and constant regular change with regard to the whole"; but the actual participants, the individuals, are only "accidentally" involved (22, n. 1531, p. 344). Accident or chance can hardly be subjected to moral judgment. However, the time of death is today determined not so much by chance as by other knowable, controllable factors. Among mortality statistics, some of the most dramatic—because of the numbers involved and the association of death with the creation of life—are those that reveal how each year some 600 thousand women die and 18 million are left handicapped or chronically ill (throughout the world, but mainly in Africa and Asia) as a result of pregnancy and childbirth. In the developed countries, these figures have been approaching zero for some time now (23, p. 12). Pluralism and equity also imply the creation of equal or similar opportunities for life whenever they are amenable to possible human action.

POPULATION AND RESOURCES:
HOW CAN INTERVENTION BE ETHICAL?

Even when society and its institutions do not intervene to ensure such opportunities for life, they at least have a passive responsibility. In the field of procreation, on the other hand, the state and the law sometimes intervene actively to constrain individuals to make pronatal or antenatal decisions. Although there is a widely shared negative moral judgment in certain cases such as selective sterilization, a much more complex and controversial issue is that concerning populations and the ethics of public choices. This is a macroethical issue, encapsulated in the question, "to what extent, using which methods, and for which purposes can the state intervene to ensure a (true or imagined) demographic balance in the ratio between resources, territory, and population?" Historically, philosophers and public authorities have adopted diverging or opposing stances on this issue, always justifying their claims by *raison d'état*. "In the ideal city-state imagined by Plato in his Laws," writes William Petersen, "the population was to be kept stable by encouraging or restricting fertility, or else by means of infanticide" (24). Aristotle also believed that neglect of this need would certainly plunge the citizens of the city-state into poverty, and that poverty was the root of evil and sedition (25). Conversely, during the period of the Empire, Rome was strongly pronatal because of both the alarming weakening of families' ties and the declining birth rate in the city. Augustus promulgated laws to punish celibacy and adultery and to reward prolific couples.

In the following centuries, the world population rose or fell for the most part spontaneously, but also as a result of human actions, such as the waging of war. The world's increase in population began to accelerate only after the Middle Ages. Because of this relative stability of world population, the "demographic question" was for centuries no longer at the focus of political and theoretical interest. Only two thousand years after Plato and Aristotle, in the late eighteenth century, a period of technological innovation and social and political change, was the need to limit births envisaged—this time for economic reasons. The risk Thomas Robert Malthus described was that of population imbalance, due, as he wrote in the first few lines of his *Essay on the Principle of Population,* "to a single great cause, closely related to man's nature: the constant tendency, inherent in all living beings, to multiply faster than the available means of subsistence will allow" (26, p. 3). Since the poor multiply faster than members of other economic classes and have fewer resources, one of the fundamental measures recommended by Malthus was, as we know, "gradually abolishing the poor laws" that provided them with public aid supplied through the parishes. According to Malthus, this aid was a more harmful and costly system than the national debt itself (26, pp. 492–493):

> For this purpose I would propose a law that parish help be denied to children
> born out of marriage contracted one year after the promulgation of this law,

and to all illegitimate children born two years after the same time. In order that this law become universally known and to engrave it more deeply in people's minds, the ministers of religion would be asked to read immediately after publication a short instruction illustrating the exact way, the strong obligation, for each man to feed his own children; the temerity and immorality of those who marry without having the means to perform such a sacred duty; the evils that have overcome the poor themselves whenever they have vainly tried to supplement, through public charity, the offices imposed by nature on the parents; and lastly the need to desist from any such claim, which had produced effects directly opposed to the purpose of those that had conceived of it.

Adam Smith followed a completely different approach to the needs of the poor in his *Wealth of Nations*. But Malthus's book and his ideas were to have a much greater influence on political decisions in nineteenth-century Europe, especially after the Restoration (cited in 27). Malthus's destiny was an odd one (although this may be an arbitrarian hypothesis) in the decades following publication of his book (1798): that of living to see his social recommendations applied and his demographic theories disproved by the facts. The development of industry and capitalism (and of its extra-European corollary, colonialism) took place almost in the absence of social rules and moral restraints, at least until the early decades of the nineteenth century; but Malthus's fundamental hypothesis, that population increases geometrically, was disproved by the facts. Though the European population grew much faster than during the eighteenth century and almost doubled (954 million in 1800; 1,654 million in 1900), the growth of resources easily outstripped it. One of the variants Malthus did not take into account in calculating the production of goods was technological innovation.

However, many have claimed, with some justification, that Malthus got his cultural revenge in the second half of the twentieth century. At this time the demographic problem of the resources/population ratio reached acute and sometimes dramatic proportions, and thus could not be neglected when making public decisions. Proponents of two main schools of thought have argued their views in recent decades on both the causes and proposed solutions: those who advocate giving priority to birth control, and those who claim that underdevelopment is a consequence rather than a cause of high birth rate and that a reduction of birth rate will result from economic and cultural growth.

On the whole it may be said that, until 1994, the prevailing trend in the world, strongly supported by the Anglo-Saxon countries, was to suggest and occasionally to impose contraception as the main, and sometimes only, remedy for the imbalance between population and resources. This policy was initially opposed by religious institutions, feminist movements, nongovernmental organizations, and the governments of some southern countries, on different and often contradictory grounds. In 1994, following a long and laborious run-up, the International Conference on Population and Development, promoted by the United

Nations, was held in Cairo, with 184 countries participating. The conference concluded with the adoption of a 20-year action program, with progress to be verified every five years. This plan, which represents a break with earlier policy, can be summarized as follows (23, pp. 1–2).

> The Program recognizes the interrelationships between consumption and production patterns, economic development, access to education, population growth, demographic structure, and environmental degradation. It emphasizes the importance of empowering women and ensuring gender equality and equity. It asserts the reciprocal relation between rights; that is, that respect for human rights is a prerequisite for the enjoyment of the highest attainable standard of health, and conversely, that the right to control every aspect of one's health and sexuality forms an important basis for the enjoyment of other rights. It puts aside demographic targets to focus on the needs and rights of individual women and men, and promotes a comprehensive reproductive health approach. It recognizes that men must take responsibility for their sexual behavior, and that their full involvement in reproductive health and child rearing is crucial. It addresses the need to provide adolescents with appropriate information and services, and includes important commitments to reduce infant and child mortality.

Of the main innovations in the five years that followed, deriving from the remainder of the "Cairo + 5" provisions completed in 1999, two should be emphasized. First, in a large number of countries, speeches on population policies switched from imperatives concerning demographic decrease to statements focusing on health (28). Second, women now play an extremely important role, both through their movements, which have contributed more than anything else to changing international culture and ethics (albeit still insufficiently), and as persons who are the main beneficiaries of an infinite number of micro-improvements in individual situations.

Examining and discussing these conditions in geographic terms would imply a focus for many bioethical issues that in reality vary profoundly worldwide (and even within the same country) and would require an analysis of the still largely unsettled scientific, ethical, and religious controversies centered on these problems (on the ethical premises and various answers to the question, "Is there a population problem?" see 29; see also 11, pp. 451–482). In view of the impossibility of carrying out this analysis to the full, I shall merely make three points.

The first point, which may appear mischievous, is that the warning given by Malthus was not exactly *there are too many of us!* but, rather, *there are too many of you!* He addressed it to the poor of the British Isles, after which his warning was sounded on a larger scale during the second half of the twentieth century with reference to the poor of the world. Whether this interpretation is considered tendentious or realistic, one cannot deny or underestimate the imbalance in many parts of the world between resources, environment, and population. In this connection I would like to add, to those I listed at the beginning of this chapter, another case of semantic hypocrisy. In international statistics and political jargon, a binary distinction is made between "developed countries" and "developing countries." However, to reflect the real state of affairs, the latter would have to be further subdivided into three groups: the true *developing* countries, those that are *at a standstill* or *stagnating* at a low level, and those that are *regressing*. This would eliminate the illusion that development is already a universal phenomenon, help spread awareness of true conditions in the "developing countries," and act as a possible stimulus for more effective actions within or on behalf of stagnating or regressing countries. The primary need, now generally acknowledged by international organizations, is not to isolate the demographic factor from its broader context but, rather, to act on each factor involved in the imbalance on the basis of valid ethical principles and extensively shared rules and procedures.

The second consideration refers precisely to ethical principles. Donald Warwick has listed these as five points, the last of which—inform, tell the truth—I have already dealt with. The other four may be summed up as follows (29):

> *Life* heads the list, for without it, people cannot benefit from the other four principles. Life means not only being alive, but enjoying good health and having reasonable security against the actions of others that cause death, illness, severe pain, or disability. *Freedom* is the capacity and opportunity to make reflective choices and to act on those choices. Freedom requires knowledge about the choices available . . . a chance to make choices without coercion or strong pressure from others . . . and the possibility of taking action to carry out the choices made. *Welfare* means a standard of living adequate to provide food, clothing, housing, health care, and education. Population programs, therefore, should not aim only to raise or lower fertility, reduce mortality, or control migration, but to be instruments for promoting human welfare. *Fairness* refers to an equitable distribution of the benefits and harms from population policies. It does not require an equal distribution of benefits and harms, but it does demand that one individual or group should not receive disproportionate advantages or disadvantages from a given policy.

My third point is that those who, like me, basically agree with these ideas should underline the existence of alternative methods. Often, for example, political choices have been based on compulsory contraception rather than on free choice, persuasion, and convenience. One of the most dramatic histories of this is in India, where a sterilization campaign was conducted in 1975 through 1977, driven by financial incentives and other rewards as well as by other forms of pressure. The result was widespread rebellion and was one of the causes of Prime Minister Indira Gandhi's downfall, as her government promoted the measures. Conversely, in many other countries, voluntary forms of birth control accompanying cultural and economic development have proved very effective, gaining wide approval from the population. Experience shows above all that the regulation of fertility can be achieved all the more rapidly and consistently when women's rights and contributions to society are recognized, especially when girls receive the necessary education—their increased freedom brings with it greater responsibility and improved options.

When the object of concern is a low rather than a high birth rate, perhaps the most effective solution, although difficult to apply, is the one proposed by Livi Bacci: "to increase confidence in life projects." How many people contemplating the bringing of a child into this world now find themselves asking, among many other, similar questions, "into what kind of world?" Perhaps we should worry less about embryos and "artificial" births and more about the naturally born, who from the beginning of their independent lives have to cope with the problems caused by those preceding them. In almost every country, the next generation will have to pay back a large share of public indebtedness, for the duration of their natural lives, as well as share in the environmental liability, a deficit that is even higher and less reversible. If we made greater efforts to help them face the mounting difficulties they will encounter as they grow up, there would be greater confidence in the future and, therefore, a higher birth rate. However, I observe that bioethics shows as little interest in this situation as does politics.

EQUITY AND POWER

I have mentioned cacothanasia, deaths that are bad in that they are predictable and avoidable, and perhaps there is no better subject for the purpose of introducing the third issue after human rights and pluralism: that of equity. Cacothanasia is unevenly distributed among individuals and peoples. Ever since the turn of the twentieth century, when Jacques Bertillon documented *inegalité sociale devant la mort* as a phenomenon simultaneously observable in Paris, Berlin, and Vienna (30), numerous studies have confirmed that this inequality exists everywhere, to a greater or lesser degree, depending on the period and the country (for Italy, see 31). (The number of such studies has increased rapidly over the past decade, although I do not know whether this is due to the greater differences in mortality rates or to researchers' increased awareness thereof.) Inequality persists despite medical progress and broader-based health services, because of a variety of interrelated factors, such as income, nutrition, housing, "lifestyle," environmental hazards, and working conditions, together with other, more specific factors. Without giving any statistical references, which are easily obtainable, I shall examine this phenomenon linked to inequality in health, partly because it is a topic with which I am familiar but, above all, because of its strong and obvious implications in the overall picture of problems related to material life. In many instances, a distinction between good and evil is difficult to make. This is usually not so, however, in choices between life and death.

In some areas (such as income) it is at least theoretically possible to pursue equality, and in others (such as justice) equality has been universally sought, at least in the realm of legislation, but the achievement of equality in length and quality of life is obviously unattainable. Nor would such an objective be desirable. To pursue it would mean standardizing the human species and canceling out the intrinsic value of differences among individuals. For this reason, although it is correct to use the term "inequality" for descriptive purposes in statistics, "inequity" is more commonly employed with reference to ethics in political choices. The latter term refers to differences that are avoidable and unnecessary, differences that must be considered unfair in the overall context of etiological knowledge and social relationships (32). In other words, the concept of equity in health implies that all individuals should have a reasonable opportunity to attain their hoped-for life potential and, more practically, that no one should be at a disadvantage in seeking such a goal if this can be avoided (33).

The obstacles to be overcome are numerous and change according to time and place. Any choices made to promote equity in health must satisfy the three criteria pointed out by Sonnino for demographic policies as a whole: universality, operability of social structures, and the active role of citizens (34, 35). This entails improving not only specific services on which health partly depends but also, more importantly, the other major factors affecting health, such as education, employment, environment, general level of equity, and social solidarity, starting from a detailed study and dissemination of the knowledge on which the personal and collective commitment of citizens can be based.

This leads us to three very brief considerations on the function of democracy in demographic choices. First, although it is clear that population policies require the application of moral principles based on knowledge and prediction, experience shows that even when this information is available it is frequently disregarded. In addition, in recent years, financial and institutional matters have gained such prominence in politics as to overshadow literally vital problems. Sometimes vital problems are viewed only as financial variables and their intrinsic value is ignored. Thus, health is treated primarily in terms of cost, just as the elderly are treated merely as the beneficiaries of pensions. A change in political outlook and in the underlying value system can ensure that population policies (including some policies not specifically intended as such that affect populations significantly) will not remain a mere addendum to decisions about the future but will accompany and to a certain extent precede such decisions.

Second, this tendency is accompanied by a strong power imbalance at the international level. Power has gradually shifted away from the United Nations and its agencies, which, at least initially, represented the world population as a whole, towards a group of governments (indicated by the acronyms G7 and G8) and to international monetary institutions. One of the most telling examples is the weakening of the World Health Organization in favor of the World Bank, which now actually directs health policy, especially in the less developed countries (36). It seems only fitting that the United Nations and its agencies, in addition to promoting international conferences on pertinent topics (in Rio de Janeiro on the environment, in Cairo on population, in Peking on women, in Rome on food policy), should have a stronger role in the actual decision-making processes.

The third consideration concerns one of the intrinsic limits of representative democracy. Certainly, more than any other system, representative democracy allows the affirmation of human rights and pluralism, as well as the pursuit of equity. However, its focus is the existing adult voting population. It does not, and hardly could, include young people in its rules, although some efforts have been made in this direction—both reasonable, such as lowering the voting age, and less reasonable, such as giving more votes to those with several children. Above all, it cannot represent the interests of a constituency of even greater size—that is, of posterity, whose interests may be, and in some cases already have been, jeopardized by our decisions. I can see no juridical remedy for this situation, except perhaps the introduction of legal norms prescribing preliminary evaluation and public discussion of the possible future impact of today's projects on health, the environment (in many countries such regulations already exist, although only with local jurisdiction), and the population. Rather than entrusting this commitment in favor of future generations to law, we should entrust it to moral evolution, which can be used as a guide in making political decisions. "If the productive sphere has penetrated the domain of action that counts," writes Hans Jonas, "so ethics must penetrate the productive sphere from which it was once excluded, and it must do so in the form of a public policy" (37).

REFERENCES

1. Reich, W. T. (ed.). *Encyclopedia of Bioethics.* Simon & Schuster, New York, 1995.
2. Graunt, J. *Natural and political observations upon the bills of mortality.* In *Les causes de la mort: Histoire naturelle et facteurs de risque,* edited by A. Fagot-Largeault. Librairie philosophique J. Vrin and Institut interdisciplinaire d'études épistémologiques, Paris-Lyon, 1989.
3. World Health Organization. *The State of World Health.* Geneva, 1995.
4. Maccararo, G. A. *Per una medicina da rinnovare. Scritti* 1966, p. 181. Feltrinelli, Milan, 1979.
5. Figà Talamanca, I. *I tossici ambientali e lavorativi e la riproduzione umana.* Piccin, Padua, 1994.
6. Ash, A. Prenatal diagnosis and selective abortion: A challenge to practice and policy. *Am. J. Public Health* 89(11): 1649–1657, 1999.
7. Berlinguer, G. Exogenous and endogenous mortality. In *Démographie: analyse et synthése,* edited by G. Caselli, J. Vallin, and G. Wunsche. 2001, in press.
8. Omenn, G. S., and Motulsky, A. G. Genetics and environment in human health. In *Encyclopedia of Bioethics,* edited by W. T. Reich, pp. 940–946. Simon & Schuster, New York, 1995.
9. Farr, W. *Vital Statistics: A Memorial Volume,* edited by N. Humphreys. Sanitary Institute of Great Britain, London, 1885.
10. Warwick, D. W. Normative approaches [under the entry Population Ethics]. In *Encyclopedia of Bioethics,* edited by W. T. Reich. Simon & Schuster, New York, 1995.

11. De Sandre, P. Demografia, politica ed etica. In *Demografia*, edited by M. Livi Bacci, G. C. Blanciardo, and A. Golini, p. 10. Fondazione Agnelli, Turin, 1994.
12. Kant, I. Per la pace perpetua: Un progetto filosofico di Immanuel Kant [1795]. In *Scritti di storia, politica e diritto*, pp. 177–178. Laterza, Bari, 1995.
13. Gaines, A. D. Race and racism. In *Encyclopedia of Bioethics*, edited by W. T. Reich, vol. 4, pp. 2189–2201. Simon & Schuster, New York, 1995.
14. Gould, S. J. *Intelligenza e pregiudizio: Le pretese scientifiche del razzismo*, pp. 209–220. Editori Riuniti, Rome, 1985. (*The Mismeasure of Man*, 1981).
15. Cavalli Sforza, L. *Geni, popoli e lingue*. Adelphi, Milan, 1996.
16. Berlinguer, G. *I flussi migratori in Italia: aspetti giuridici ed etici, relazione*. Congresso nazionale di Igiene, Naples, September 26, 1996.
17. Golini, A. Foreword. In *Tendenze demografiche e politiche per la popolazione: Terzo Rapporto IRP*, edited by A. Golini, p. 10. Il Mulino, Bologna, 1994.
18. De Vincentiis, G., and Lauricella, E. Necessité di una urgente revisions della legislazione e dei regolamenti in campo ostetrico-ginecologico. Paper presented at the Congress of the Società italiana di ostetricia e ginecologia, Rome, 1968.
19. Kant, I. Sul detto comune: questo può essere giusto in teoria, ma non vale per la prassi. In *Scritti di storia, politica e diritto*, pp. 122–161. Laterza, Bari, 1995.
20. Rodotà, S. *Tecnologie e diritti*. Il Mulino, Bologna, 1995.
21. Veca, S. *Etica e politica. I dilemmi del pluralismo: democrazia reale e democrazia possible*, p. 22. Garzanti, Milan, 1989.
22. Leopardi, G. *Zibaldone*. Newton, Rome, 1997.
23. Girard, F. Cairo + five: Reviewing progress for women. *J. Women's Health Law* 1(1), 1999.
24. Petersen, W. History of population: Theories. In *Encyclopedia of Bioethics*, edited by W. T. Reich, p. 1962. Simon & Schuster, New York, 1995.
25. Aristotle. *La politica*, 2.9.
26. Malthus, T. R. *Saggio sul principio di popolazione*. Utet, Turin, 1965 (*An Essay on the Principle of Population as It Affects the Future Improvement of the Society*, London, 1798).
27. Rothschild, E. Social security and laissez-faire in the eighteenth century political economy. *Popul. Dev. Rev.* 21(4): 711–744, 1995.
28. Correa, S., and Sen, G. Cairo + 5: Avanzare nell'occhio del cyclone. In *Social Watch*, pp. 85–90. Osservatorio internazionale sullo sviluppo sociale. Rosenberg & Sellier, Turin, 1999.
29. Warwick, D. P. Elements of population ethics. In *Encyclopedia of Bioethics*, edited by W. T. Reich, vol. 4, pp. 1956–1962. Simon & Schuster, New York, 1995.
30. Bertillon, J. Mouvements de popoulation et causes de décès selon le degré d'aisance a Paris, Berlin, Vienee. In *Proceedings of the 10th International Hygiene and Demography Congress*, p. 961. Paris, 1900.
31. Costa, G., and Faggiano, F. *L'equità nella salute in Italia*. Franco Angeli, Milan, 1994.
32. Whitehead, M. *The Concepts and Principles of Equity and Health*. WHO Regional Office for Europe, Copenhagen, 1990.
33. World Health Organization. *Social Justice and Equity in Health*. Report of a WHO meeting. WHO Regional Office for Europe, Copenhagen, 1986.

34. Dahlgren, G., and Whitehead, M. *Policies and Strategies to Promote Equity in Health.* WHO Regional Office for Europe, Copenhagen, 1992.
35. Sonnino, E. *Aspetti e problemi di demografia sociale e di politica della popolazione in Italia,* pp. 58–65. Istituto di demografia dell'Università di Roma, Rome, 1979.
36. Berlinguer, G. Globalization and global health. *Int. J. Health Serv.* 29(3): 579–595, 1999.
37. Jonas, H. *Il principio responsabilità,* p. 14. Einaudi, Turin, 1990.

CHAPTER 3

Work And Health:
Foundations And Ethical Conflicts

ETHICS AND BUSINESS

The relationship between work and health lies at the interface between human biology and economics, that is, between two fields in which the interest in ethics is growing. That bioethics should be involved was only to be expected, as it grew out of increased knowledge of and progress in the biomedical sciences. It was, perhaps, less to be expected that Mr. John Shad, president of the Securities and Exchange Commission, the U.S. financial market's watchdog organization, should have donated $30 million to the Harvard Business School to establish a new teaching subject, Ethics and Business. G. Rossi, Mr. Shad's counterpart in Italy, wrote in *Corriere della sera,* the Fiat-owned daily, "The problem of the relationship between ethics and business activities has always been a cause of the most anguished soul-searching in ancient and modern thought. It becomes topical whenever a period of crisis or transition occurs. . . . Proclamations about ethics are a sign that something is wrong with Western economy or that law is in crisis, and so times are ripe for radical reforms of the system" (1). If this is true for Western economies, it is all the more true for the rest of the world, which Western economic forces influence so profoundly.

It is within this framework that we must conduct our moral reflections on the relationship between work and health, which was rarely a substantial part of the "anguished soul-searching in . . . ancient thought." It may be of interest to examine this relationship in outline, in order to evaluate how new topics, ideas, interests, and subjects have emerged in recent times: economy and society, capital and labor, politics and institutions, laws and moral rules. In this field we find many ethical conflicts among different values, sometimes mutually antagonistic and sometimes reconcilable, each with its own practical validity and moral legitimacy: a typical example, one of the more significant and stimulating, of the difficulty of (and need for) ethical reflection in a complex society.

55

BERNARDINO RAMAZZINI: THE ETHICS OF VIRTUE

One possible chronological and methodological starting point, since moral stimuli often influence scientists' choices, might be to examine the reasons that led Bernardino Ramazzini, in 1700, to write *Diseases of Workers* (2), the first treatise on this topic, which contains accurate, often anguished descriptions of the techniques and pathologies associated with some 41 occupations (plus 12 more in the following edition). Ramazzini's motivations are clearly stated in his introduction to the first edition of the book and may be interpreted as based on two virtues. The first of these is compassion, the Latin *pietas:* suffering together, the shared feeling of humanity, which is one of the earliest roots of medical ethics. As well as extending to individual patients, Ramazzini's compassion extends to the vast category of all those who work, whatever their occupation: "We must admit that workers in some arts and crafts sometimes derive from them grave injuries, so that where they hoped for a subsistence that would prolong their lives and feed their families, they are too often repaid with the most dangerous diseases and, finally, uttering curses on the profession to which they had devoted themselves, they desert their place among the living. When I was engaged in the practice of medicine, I observed that this very often happens. And so I have tried my utmost to compose a special treatise on the disease of the workers" (2). David Hume, several decades later, wrote that "pity depends largely on the contiguity or indeed the sight of the object" (3). Ramazzini set out to document and disclose a harsh, previously hidden reality in order to arouse feelings that would move society to relieve the suffering of workers.

The other virtue is gratitude, the acknowledgment due to those who have benefited us with their work. As Ramazzini writes, "We owe this [the book] to the wretched conditions of the workers, from whose manual toil, so necessary though sometimes very mean and sordid, so many benefits accrue to the commonwealth of mankind [in the original, *humanae reipublicae*]; yes, this debt must be paid by the most glorious of all the arts, as Hippocrates calls it in his *Precepts,* that of Medicine, which cures without a fee and succors the poor" (2, p. 9). In his praise of medicine, Ramazzini is careful also to add some criticism and even a few ironic remarks, as in the chapter on the diseases of *corpse bearers,* free men forced by the harsh conditions of poverty to undertake these wretched functions, whose fate is strongly to be pitied because of the serious diseases to which they are prone. And yet, he says, "it is only fair, seeing that they bury in the earth not only the dead but the doctor's mistakes as well, that the art of medicine should do them a good turn and repay them for saving the reputation of the profession."

Ramazzini doubtless had additional motivations in writing his book—in the first instance, the thirst for scientific knowledge that characterized the seventeenth century and an explicit desire to contribute, at a time when the scientific and mechanical arts were developing, both to the good of the state and to the relief of the worker (*artificum*). However, we cannot ignore the author's more specific motivation. This is found consistently both in the declaration of intent and in the individual chapters, in which indignation, pity, generosity, and altruism always mingle with scientific documentation. It is true that the philosophy of our century, in order to encourage a less subjective and variable analysis of ethics, has often treated virtues as secondary to an ethics based on principles and rules, devoting considerable attention to utilitarian and deontological theories and often separating the question of whether an action is right or equitable from the character of the agent and criticizing the ethics of virtue, because "its strong agent perspective prevents it from giving us sufficiently specific advice about what we ought to do" (4). The cultural good fortune and practical consequences of Ramazzini's work represent one of many demonstrations that those two needs may be reconciled.

ADAM SMITH: THE WEALTH OF NATIONS AND THE WORKERS' WELFARE

Ramazzini's work, focusing on compassion and gratitude and opening new vistas in the knowledge and prevention of disease, was immediately translated into numerous languages and was widely circulated in Europe. The facts he revealed and the concepts he developed had a strong and lasting impact. It is interesting to note, for example, that his book is cited, for the purpose of describing human suffering in the workplace, in two texts, one published in the eighteenth century, the other in the nineteenth. Both of these works, Adam Smith's *An Enquiry into the Nature and Causes of the Wealth of Nations* (published in 1776) and Karl Marx's *Das Kapital* (vol. I, published in 1867), became classics in the canons of otherwise differing schools of thought and have had a profound influence on economic theory and social action over the past centuries.

Adam Smith quotes Ramazzini, in the chapter devoted to the remuneration of work, when he states that "almost every kind of workman is subject to some peculiar infirmity due to a peculiar application to a peculiar type of work. . . . If the employers were always to listen to the dictates of reason and humanity, they would often have cause to moderate rather than stimulate the application of their workers" (5). This statement is linked to the theory that the wealth of nations requires freedom of trade and enterprise and, above all, security for all (especially the middle class)—that is, security not for the aristocracy alone but for those performing work of all kinds. A liberal remuneration of work is thus required, which is a necessary effect and natural indicator of the growing wealth of the nation. Smith refuted the idea, current at the time, that men worked better when badly nourished than when well fed, when discouraged than when in high spirits, when wages were lower (often in times of illness and death) than when they were higher.

In addition to these considerations based on profit and philanthropy ("the dictates of reason and humanity"), which led him to write that no society in which the majority of the members are poor and unhappy can flourish and be happy,

Adam Smith also introduced the concept of justice, which would have great importance in the following centuries, asserting that it is substantially fair that those who feed, clothe, and house the entire population should enjoy a part of the fruits of their labor, so that they themselves may be adequately nourished, clothed, and housed. (For an analysis of Smith's thoughts on this topic, see 6.) From these concerns, based on a common interest for society in the welfare of all its members, Smith derived the need for a legal regulation of labor relations, opening the way to what is now known as "public ethics."

THE NINETEENTH CENTURY:
LABOR BETWEEN JUSTICE AND LAISSEZ-FAIRE

The concept of justice, linked to the idea of freedom and (natural) human rights possessed by each individual as a human being, lay at the heart of two great events that changed the world at the end of the eighteenth century—the American War for Independence and defense of the right of each individual to life and liberty (as subsequently codified in the U.S. Constitution), and the French Revolution and the merging of *liberté* with *égalité*. These events engendered both recognition of the principles of freedom and human rights and the adoption of rules capable of enforcing them. We may be certain that these ideas moved peoples and changed nations, although they filtered down to the everyday life of ordinary workers with tragic slowness. We know that, for almost the entire nineteenth century, laissez-faire capitalism was accompanied by the unbridled exploitation of workers, including women and children, and took place in the absence of any set limits or rules. The consequences, widely documented by the inquiries of health inspectors, by local authorities, and by researchers sensitive to the problem, have been defined by some historians as a "peaceful genocide." The severe deterioration in living conditions, the widespread damage to health, and the precarious security of workers, starting from the early Industrial Revolution, could be read as a cynical confirmation that moral principles have little or no effect in the relief of daily suffering of human beings. I consider it more useful to analyze why and how this change in working conditions came to be.

One of the reasons is that, at the end of the eighteenth century, and in contradiction to the ideas of Adam Smith and the two revolutions, other moral principles emerged that were to be dominant until the end of the nineteenth century. Philosophies that espouse laissez-faire have always been accompanied, and justified, by ethical arguments concerning human nature, human behavior, and the task for society. In a counterargument to, for example, the principle stated by the revolutionary and social reformer Condorcet—namely, that the causes of poverty and destitution are to be sought in evil institutions, not in the laws governing human nature—Thomas Robert Malthus suggested that it was necessary to consider man as he really was: "inert, indolent and adverse to labor, unless obliged by necessity." Social justice, according to Malthus, would thus not be desirable as "the general tendency towards a uniform pathway to prosperity leads to the degradation rather than the exaltation of the character." Only need and fear, he claimed, and not compassion and gratitude, could serve as a stimulus to work and make a contribution to prosperity (7).

This kind of authoritarian paternalism, in which the judgment of what is good for a person (or a group of persons) is imposed on the subject, was accompanied in the early stages of the Industrial Revolution by the idea that the ethics of production is confined to the realm of profit; this idea was reaffirmed in 1970 by Milton Friedman in a trend-setting article, "The Responsibility of Business Is to Make Profit" (8, cited in 9). Acceptance of the moral legitimacy of this principle was rooted in the belief that the unremitting pursuit of profit would ultimately produce a benefit for the majority of the population, a belief that was for a long time widely shared and overshadowed all other ethical principles. Unfortunately, history and experience have shown that, while "free enterprise" was and still is the basis of extraordinary economic development, its accompanying ethics can be the cause of a broad and deep sacrifice of workers' health and security.

In the first half of the nineteenth century, this ethics was totally dominant. However, its consequences were subjected to profound moral scrutiny, such as that developed by Giacomo Leopardi in *Zibaldone*. He begins with the coining of currency and ultimately arrives at all the goods that are necessary for "what we call the perfection and happiness of mankind" (10):

> Observe, in the modern perfection of the arts, the immense toil and hardship that are necessary to produce money for society. Begin with the work in the mines, and the extraction of metals, and work down as far as the final operation of coining. Note how many men are forcibly subjected to regular and permanent unhappiness, to disease, death, slavery (either gratuitous or violent, or mercenary), to disaster, poverty, hardship, hard labor of every kind, in order to procure for other men this means of civilization, and presumed means of happiness. Tell me, therefore, first, whether nature can possibly have set from the outset this price to be paid by men for this perfection and happiness; that is, the price of a regular unhappiness for one-half of the men (and in saying one-half, I am not considering only this, but also other branches of so-called social perfection that cost the same price). Tell me, second, whether this wretchedness of our fellow men is consistent with this very civilization they are supposed to serve. It is well known how slavery is defended by large numbers of politicians and so on. It is retained in practice in spite of the theories, as it is deemed necessary for the comfort, the perfection, the good, the civilization of society. And what I am saying about money is true also for the food that comes to us from very distant parts by means of the same and similar hardship, slavery, etc. Like sugar, coffee, etc., etc. And that are deemed necessary for the perfection of society. And see how this, like civilization (as all false theories are wont), contradicts itself also in theory and moreover cannot exist in the absence of circumstances that are repugnant to its

nature and are absolutely uncivilized, indeed barbaric in all the truth and force of the term. So that perfect civilization cannot exist without perfect barbarity, the perfection of society without its imperfection; and once you remove this imperfection, you cut the very roots of the asserted perfection of society.

KARL MARX:
USE OR DEPREDATION OF THE WORK FORCE

As I mentioned earlier, Karl Marx also used Ramazzini as a basis for his description of workers' condition. However, he set out from the idea—and I say this without any intention to make an artificial comparison with the long extract from Leopardi above—that "a certain intellectual and physical benumbing is inseparable even from the division of labor in society as a whole." He then goes on to stress—and this is the object of his thinking—the essential point: "The period of manufacturing, by carrying this social separation of the branches of labor much further, and on the other hand corroding the very roots of the individual's life through its very peculiar division of labor, is also the first to provide the material and the stimulus for *industrial pathology*" (11, pp. 63–64), that is, the extension of the catalogue of occupational diseases described by Ramazzini.

In his analysis of wage-earning workers, Marx suggests a clear-cut distinction,with obvious ethical implications, between the use and the depredation of labor, a misuse that often dooms workers to an early death. The purchasing of workers' labor is one thing, the plundering of working capacity quite another; indeed, Marx considers working capacity as the only "good" possessed by the worker, who, in order to continue selling it, must have the possibility of replenishing it. In the long chapter he dedicates to "the working day," Marx represents the dialogue between the two antagonists as follows (11, pt. 1, pp. 254–255):

> You and I, on the market, know only one language, that of the exchange of goods. And the consumption of the goods does not pertain to the seller, who disposes of it, but to the buyer, who purchases it. The use of my daily labor pertains to you. But with its daily selling price I must daily renew it in order to go on selling it. Neglecting the natural wear and tear due to age, etc., I must be able to work tomorrow in the same normal conditions of strength, health, and freshness as today. You preach to me daily the gospel of "thrift" and "abstinence." Well, I want to administer my only capital, labor, like a reasonable and thrifty economist, and want to refrain from all insane wasting thereof. I want to make available daily, by setting it in motion and converting it into work, only as much as is compatible with its normal duration and its healthy development. You want to have at your disposal *in a single day,* by means of an unreasonable extension of the working day, a quantity of my labor exceeding that which I am able to replenish in three days. The issue of my labor and its *depredation* are two quite different matters. . . . I therefore demand a working day of *normal* length, and I demand it without appealing to your heart, because in money matters feelings are no longer involved. You

may be a model citizen, perhaps a member of the League for the abolition of cruelty to animals, and perhaps even in odor of sanctity, but the thing you represent before me has no heart beating in its breast. . . . I demand a *normal working day* because I demand the value of my goods, like any other seller.

The conclusion of the argument is that in the regulation of the labor relationship, "an antinomy occurs: right against right"; for this reason, "in the history of capitalistic production *the regulation of the working day* is presented as a *struggle to set the limits of the working day*—a struggle between the collective capitalist, that is, *the class of capitalists,* and the collective worker, that is, *the working class*" (11, pt. 1, p. 255).

I should like to add to this argument a comment on its field of application in later periods. Marx's argument began from the point of greatest conflict in the second half of the nineteenth century—the number of working hours. The conflict directly concerned *the working day,* which had been extended out of all proportion, and, indirectly, other forms of extension of working time: from the use of minors, to the "porosity" of work, down to the reduction in the number of rest days (including religious holidays, which led Paul Lafargue, Marx's son-in-law, to assert in his *Droit à la paresse* that Protestantism, as a "Christian religion adapted to suit the new industrial and commercial needs of the middle class, had fewer scruples about popular rest days: it dethroned the saints in heaven in order to abolish their feast days on earth" (12)). However, the field of application of the argument was extended by Marx (and greatly by others after Marx) beyond the question of working hours to embrace every aspect of work liable to cause damage, wear and tear, and depredation of workers' health and longevity, as the effects of environment, materials and products, work rate, and so forth were gradually recognized. These aspects of work, too, logically became objects of dispute in the confrontation and, often, opposition—rights against rights—that marked labor relations in many countries in the late nineteenth and most of the twentieth century.

MORAL PROGRESS AND MATERIAL CONDITIONS

The way in which this contradiction between philosophies was faced through struggle or cooperation between labor and capital, together with the progress made in production techniques, legislation, and ethical ideas, had a marked effect on the history of the health and safety of workers over the past hundred years. The history of the conflict may be interpreted in the light of different experiences and points of view, and the degree to which these vary accounts for the differences worldwide (between, for instance, America and Europe) based on particular cultures, rules, and the influence of workers' movements. The variations among areas can be used to analyze the diachronic developments and the ethical values that contributed to the successes and failures of prevention programs. We can also discuss both the ethical bases of the behavior characterizing the different situations and the different actions undertaken by the many interested parties: capital and labor, the state and the law, religion and politics, technology and science, medicine and the new professions.

The main positive phenomenon is that, throughout this history, workers' material conditions, particularly in the developed countries, have improved substantially. The ethical evaluation of labor has been both transformed and enhanced. Work is no longer universally considered a biblical curse, something to be tolerated as a consequence of divine will or immutable human laws, but considered a right, which may become an avenue for the expression of freedom and creativity. In some cases work has even been used as a means to help the disabled, to integrate them in many activities and allow them to develop their own personalities. All this represents a reversal of the historically negative nature of both image and substance in the relation between work and the integrity of body and mind.

The principle of justice, however, is endangered by the huge distance that separates these possibilities from everyday reality. I should like to emphasize two facts. The first is the existence, or increase, of inequalities in health and safety between the different social classes (according to occupation) in the developed countries, as has been clearly documented where not ignored or distorted through manipulation of a country's vital statistics. The gap between life expectancy at the two extremes (unskilled manual workers and professionals and managers) ranges from five to ten years everywhere; moreover, it persists, although to a lesser degree, even where prevention of specific diseases and accidents and equal access to health care are practiced. Today, in the developed countries, this gap is due not so much to specific causes (toxic substances, fatigue, accidents) as to psychosocial causes: disparities in income, education, self-respect, stress, autonomy, organization of work, gratification obtained from work—in essence, everything implied in recognizing oneself and being recognized, a necessity that Adam Smith identified in *The Theory of Moral Sentiments* as the prime need of every individual and was the basis of his ethics grounded on sympathy (13). The second fact is that, as we endeavor to investigate bioethical issues of the technological and scientific present—in some cases, perhaps, more of the future than the present—we see with anguish that in many countries the most ancient and inhuman exploitation not only persists but is actually spreading. I am referring to slavery and bondage, working practices that have been morally rejected for centuries and declared illegal by the Slavery Convention of 1926, as promulgated by the League of Nations.

ETHICAL AND MORAL TENDENCIES

In recent decades, the moral principles associated with the relationship between human work, economics, and health have on occasion been clearly and authoritatively defined. For the sake of example, I refer here to three different sources.

One is the Encyclical *Pacem in terris,* issued in 1963, by Pope John XXIII (14). The chapter entitled "Rights Relevant To The Economic World" begins with the following statements:

> 17. Human beings have the inherent right to free enterprise in the economic field and the right to work.
> 18. These rights are inextricably linked to the right to working conditions that are not harmful to physical health and morality and do not hinder the integral development of the human beings being trained and, in the case of women, to the right to working conditions compatible with their needs and duties as wives and mothers.

The second source is the *Declaration on Workers' Health,* issued in 1992, by eminent authorities from the worlds of economics, politics, and science, meeting under the auspices of the Pan-American Health Organization during the year dedicated by PAHO to safety and health in the workplace (15). After emphasizing "the high cost of disability and loss of life due to work-related diseases and unhealthy working conditions, including conditions of serious risk, that could be eliminated and controlled," the declaration goes on to emphasize two ethical aspects of the relationship between work and health:

> The aims of economic progress are only justified to the extent that concern is focused on human beings and their social well-being, and that in order to ensure viable and sustained growth it is essential that workers enjoy good levels of health. Knowledge is available about the strategies and techniques for reducing, eliminating, and controlling occupational risk factors; the application of this knowledge is not only beneficial for workers, but also leads to the attainment of a more equitable, stable, and productive society.

The third source directly concerns professionals working in this field. In 1992, the International Commission on Occupational Health (ICOH), after numerous consultations, published an *International Code of Ethics for Occupational Health Professionals* comprising 26 paragraphs (16). The ICOH summed up its significant points as follows:

> 1. Occupational health practice must be performed according to highest professional standards and ethical principles. Occupational health professionals must serve the health and social well-being of the workers, individually and collectively. They must also contribute to environmental and community health.
> 2. The obligations of occupational health professionals include protecting the life and health of the workers, respecting human dignity, and promoting the highest ethical principles in occupational health policies and programs. Integrity in professional conduct, impartiality, and the protection of the confidentiality of health data and of the privacy of the workers are part of these obligations.
> 3. Occupational health professionals are experts who must enjoy full professional independence in the execution of their functions. They must acquire

and maintain the competence necessary for their duties, and require conditions which allow them to carry out their tasks according to good practice and professional ethics.

The conclusions represented in the above extracts—the first from a religious source, the second from an institutional source, the third from a professional source—appear, on the whole (with some exceptions, to which I shall return later), straightforward and convergent. Nevertheless, scientific progress, the laws of the market, civil and penal legislation, and the code of ethics of the health professions do not provide up-to-date responses to the ethical problems that arise in many aspects of modern work. I am referring in particular to the conflicts between different values and interests, each of which has its own legitimate justification.

I can understand that choosing an approach to investigation of this issue that involves pointing out these conflicts may elicit some objections, particularly because other possible paths could be followed. For example, one might take a historical path, looking at technological developments or ethical ideas that changed substantially during slavery and during the Industrial Revolution, particularly after workers were acknowledged as having rights of their own. Another approach might be to follow the threads of several typical concepts of the relationship between health and work, such as hazards and the relationship between costs and benefits. Or, again, one might explore how the various schools of bioethical thought have treated this topic. I prefer to start with the conflicts because they actually exist; because, even though these conflicts have often been given an ideological interpretation, they relate to different material interests and moral subjects; and, lastly, because the only way to understand and then to accept, overcome, or resolve conflicts is to acknowledge them.

We can perhaps take as the basis for our approach—making all due distinctions about the differing times and context—the fifth thesis of Immanuel Kant, regarding his ideas on universal history: "the greatest problem of mankind, to solve which it is forced by nature, is the attainment of a civil society in which law is universally acknowledged," which has as its starting point "a general antagonism among its members but at the same time the most rigorous determination and assurance of the limits of such a freedom, so that it can coexist with the freedom of others" (17).

In particular, in mixing (sometimes arbitrarily, I fear) an exposition of the facts with moral evaluations, I refer to the following points, each of which makes up a section of this chapter:

1. Conflict between the right of workers to life, health, and safety and the right of enterprises to maximize production
2. Conflicts related to information: the right of workers to be informed of risks, the right of enterprises to industrial and commercial secrecy, and the rights and duties of professional experts

3. Conflicts between production and the external environment, between workers and population
4. Conflicts among workers
5. Conflicts between work and reproductive health, including childbirth

WORKERS AND ENTERPRISES

The Selection (Genetic or Other) of Workers

There has always been a conflict between the health and safety needs of workers and the tendency of enterprises to pursue maximum production at minimum costs. The form of this conflict has changed according to the period and the society, and is not resolved even when public ownership replaces private ownership of the enterprise. The relationship between the values and interests of workers and enterprises, values and interests that occasionally coincide but are usually contradictory, has normally been regulated according to four factors: (*a*) what has been brutally (but realistically) defined as the "power ratio" between the social partners, (*b*) the laws of the state, (*c*) technological development, and (*d*) ethical principles.

One of the most important new aspects in these relations is that the regulation of dealings between workers and enterprises, in addition to the factors listed above, is increasingly influenced by scientific knowledge, its technological applications, and the function of specialists who take part in the decision-making. Previously based on empirical evaluations, many decisions now pass through this filter.

One typical example is the selection of the workers at the time of hiring and during periodic evaluations. Hiring was once performed informally, with the company representative judging a group of hopeful workers and selecting those most suitable for the task with a casual wave of his hand; this was the case for both laborers in the village square and dock workers at the port. Over the last century, evaluations have gradually been based on the methods of specialists: first, the medical visit; then aptitude testing, psychosocial assessment, and behavior tests; and, later, more complex systems involving genetics, the identification of subjects hypersensitive to certain hazards, predictive medicine, biological monitoring of workers, and evaluation of conditions and behaviors outside the workplace liable to increase risk and absence from work (obesity, smoking, lack of exercise).

In recent times, bioethical discussion has focused on genetic screening, a new frontier of science and ethics, ignoring other forms of selection. For example, some companies have applied a "reverse selection" process, in which less suitable or less capable subjects—for example, minors, weaker ethnic groups, or immigrants—are hired for the simple reason that they are more defenseless. But employers justify the range of selection techniques with one argument: the company must determine who is capable of performing a given task.

Three ethical problems arise in the field of selection, which Thomas H. Murray, one of the first to tackle this issue, has summed up as follows. First, what are the implications of the power imbalance in the employer-employee relationship for issues of justice? Second, what limits should exist on what an employer can know about its employees? Third, how much influence should an employer have over its employees' behavior outside work (18, p. 1848; see also 19)? The answers have become more complex in recent decades as the range of assessments has been extended. No longer merely establishing whether workers are able to perform their tasks competently, evaluators seek to forecast the degree of risk to which workers are prone for occupational and non-occupational pathologies.

The ethical problems accompanying employee health screenings arise in different ways, depending on a country's health care system. These problems are particularly evident in the United States, where health care is based on private insurance policies taken out by individuals or by companies on behalf of their employees, and where is obviously a predisposition to include or exclude a subject (or to adjust the premiums) according to the state of health or proneness to disease. Such ethical problems are less compelling or even nonexistent where health care is universal, since the costs of the system are shared among all workers or by the entire nation and are thus not a critical consideration for employers. In these arguably morally superior systems, the workers are less likely to risk not being treated and is less subject to decisions that are possibly arbitrary or are, in any case, dictated by considerations extraneous to their vital interests.

As more and more companies subject their workers to genetic screening programs, particularly in the United States (20; see also 21, cited in 22), two ethical problems arise. The first is the issue of workers' privacy. Any breach of "genetic privacy" can be very dangerous. Stefano Rodotà has written in this connection (23):

> We live in times in which the mechanisms of acceptance of what is different seem to break down at every step. But the older forms of discrimination and stigmatization, which led people to rail against drug addicts, homosexuals, and Communists, are likely to be dramatically surpassed by the over-emphasis given to genetic diversity. Those who used to be the object of these vile accusations were in any case allowed a chance to redeem themselves: treatment for addiction, sexual abstinence, ideological abjuration. This possibility does not exist in the case of genetic diversity, which is independent of the individual's will; which pertains to the deep structure of a person; which is a mark of destiny, not a choice. The condemnation is thus likely to be without appeal.

To quote a remark by J. Harris, it is likely that "workers identified as being 'at risk' are worried about their condition and the consequences deriving from it, and that this situation of anguish could continue for the rest of their lives, which may prove to be long and healthy" (24).

The second ethical problem concerns the screening of workers with regard to the hazards of particular work environments, a type of screening increasingly in use in many countries. The main moral justification is that it benefits job seekers who, if hired, might find themselves, for example, exposed to chemical substances to which they are hypersensitive. Such screening may be necessary in certain environments, in order to protect the worker and others. However, Murray's warning that "careful scrutiny of the ethics of such policies must continue" (18, p. 1851) is justified on several grounds, that I will sum up as follows:

1. The validity of many types of predictive test has not been adequately documented; in particular, "the science of identifying genetic factors that may contribute to the onset of work-related diseases is still in its infancy" (25, p. 1845).
2. Those who are excluded from a job by screening run the risk of remaining unemployed and thus of falling ill because of this condition. In the developed countries, where health care has been established for dangerous activities, unemployment becomes the most serious "occupational disease."
3. If the system were to become generalized, only super-resistant subjects would be hired. (Probably not even Superman, as he is known to be genetically vulnerable to kryptonite.)
4. Employers who select workers based not on their skills but on enhanced resistance to harmful environmental factors can argue for a lesser need for primary preventive measures and, indeed, can represent an obstacle to the introduction of such measures. In practice, "the possibility of selecting the employees 'at risk' could reduce the obligation to make the workplace or the physical environment safe and healthy, thus making the world at large a more dangerous and unpleasant place" (24).

In the United States, too, there is growing concern over the potential for abuses in the genetic selection of employees. On February 8, 2000, President Clinton issued an Executive Order banning all forms of discrimination based on genetic information in government jobs: "It is the policy of the Government of the United States to provide equal employment opportunity in Federal employment for all qualified persons and to prohibit discrimination against employees based on the receipt of genetic services. This policy of equal opportunity applies to every aspect of Federal employment" (26). Federal employees are thus protected. And others? The issue of "two ethics" cuts across several regulatory fields in the United States.

Workers' Compensation

Compensation to workers (usually but not always monetary) for hazardous working conditions or for injuries suffered has been a commonplace in many countries for at least a century. The first compulsory insurance against occupational accidents, introduced in Bismarck's Germany (27) and subsequently the model for workers' compensation, established a dual guarantee: for firms, which were no longer sued for compensation, and for workers, who were able to obtain compensation for injuries suffered.

Italy's recent history includes an example of a novel interpretation of the idea of compensation for workers. Until the mid-1960s, it was company policy in Italy to offer (and for trade unions to demand) wage increases as compensation for hazardous conditions in the workplace. One consequence of this policy was that, with no incentive for the company to invest in improvement of working conditions, the incidence of occupational diseases increased steadily for decades and the number of accidents rose from an average of 171 cases per thousand worker-years in 1951–1955 to a maximum of 231 cases in 1963. Only in 1963 did trade unions begin negotiating for healthier and safer working environments, using the motto, "Health is not for sale" (for a reconstruction of this movement, see 28; see also 29, 30). Vigorous efforts over the next 15 years won concessions that had far-reaching effects: cases of accident and disease in the workplace fell by a third and deaths by a half; laws were enacted that stipulated that workers had the right to be informed about and to exert control over the production environment; and technological innovation was stimulated, with consequent benefits for industrial activities. Although the improvements were only temporary in many cases, with companies returning to their previous policies—offering higher pay for higher risk—Italy's experience nevertheless influenced the trade union movements and scientific environments of other countries.

I have summarized the practical effects of Italy's innovations in the field of employment compensation, but the ethical implications are quite as significant:

1. The recognition that the value of life and health is greater than the customary monetary compensation for their loss
2. The perception that economic activities "cannot be carried on in contradiction with social utility or in such a way as to be harmful to safety, freedom, or human dignity" (art. 41 of the Italian Constitution)
3. The transition from workers' thinking of themselves purely as sellers of labor to their thinking of themselves as partners in production; that is, to being informed and aware of their status as, among other roles, technological innovators
4. The construction of a model for controlling environmental conditions "from the bottom up," which grew out of working experiences and depended on the collaboration of workers and professional experts (production technicians, physicians, chemists, psychologists, etc.)

The most common kind of compensation is in the form of a payment after an unfortunate occurrence (accident, disease, hospitalization, death). The monetary damages are paid according to precisely formulated rules. Some of these rules refer to the amount of the compensation, which is based on two criteria: (*a*) the extent of damage, a usually quantifiable value; and (*b*) the monetary value assigned to physical integrity, health, and life, which is more difficult to quantify, as these values are anything but uniform. Other rules govern the procedures for the payment of damages; in Europe, the process is normally pro forma and limited to ascertaining the particulars of the event. In the United States, however, compensation often depends on the successful demonstration through legal action of a causal relationship between a specific job and the damage incurred. One of the deficiencies of the latter system has been described by Charles Levenstein: "The system does not deal effectively with occupational diseases. Workers have the burden of demonstrating that their illness is job-related. Diseases of long latency and that may have multiple causes are rarely diagnosed as occupational and workers suffering from them are rarely compensated" (31). In some cases, including those involving tumors caused by asbestos (mesothelioma of the pleura), which have a latency of up to 30 years, the counsel for the worker was able to demonstrate the necessary causal link and to obtain compensation from the industries producing and using the asbestos. However, compensation in most of these cases was posthumous.

Control of Behavior

Even when timely, workers' compensation always follows the suffering, the damage, the disease—events that are often avoidable; and it does not always result in increased efforts at prevention. But anticipating and preventing potential threats to health in the workplace does more than just limit the costs of compensation to the employer. It also tends to enhance the physical and psychological well-being of the worker, which is, of course, both an intrinsic good and a condition of individual freedom (32). In the history of prevention of occupational illness and injury, the industrial hygiene approach, based on modifying the technology, the organization, and the work environment for the benefit of all who work there, has proved more effective than protection designed for individual use, although individual protection continues to be necessary in many cases. Sometimes criticized as paternalistic in that it limits the subject's autonomy (for arguments for and against paternalism in safety regulations, see 33), industrial hygiene is justified on many practical and moral grounds.

Policies that seek to improve the health and safety of workers through control of their behavior, sometimes even outside the workplace, are more dubious. These policies have numerous precedents in history (the first labor inspectors in English factories, for example, were clergymen who were given the task of checking both the physical and moral integrity of the workers). However, efforts to control the behavior of workers have increased considerably in recent years, especially under the rubric of "health promotion," which combines individual commitment and collective action with health education and prevention. To this end, many U.S. companies have begun to offer cash incentives to workers willing to adopt healthier behavior—for example, awarding a prize to anyone who stops smoking (to be returned in the event of relapse) or rewarding each pound of weight lost by obese workers (and penalizing the worker a like amount for each pound regained). Some companies also offer incentives for engaging in physical activities such as bicycling, swimming, running, or walking, paying according to time spent or distance traveled. Through these programs, workers enjoy better health and employers reduce both health insurance expenditures and employee hours lost to illness.

It is no doubt beneficial to give up smoking, to keep your weight down, and to avoid leading a sedentary life. But imposing restrictions on workers' behavior by means of monetary incentives and more or less open coercion is debatable in practice. Granted, giving up smoking would almost certainly benefit anyone; it is not certain, however, that this is true with regard to losing weight or engaging in physical exercise or sport. Changes in diet or activity level must be made carefully, preferably with professional guidance. Otherwise there is the risk that in trying to correct one problem you create another problem—physical or psychological. But the ethical objections to employer-imposed behavioral restrictions also have implications for health.

One such objection was clearly stated by Allegrante and Sloan in an editorial published in *Preventive Medicine* (34), based on the observation that we often tend "to perceive the world as a just place, where people get what they deserve and deserve what they get." As a result, "if people become ill, we tend to attribute the cause of their illness to them and to their behavior. In this way, at least psychologically, we are protected against the possibility that we will suffer from the same illness. Following this logic, it becomes convenient to target health promotion at individuals rather than organizations, since individuals are seen to be the cause of their illness."

This perception has two consequences. One, "blaming the victim," entails condemning the sufferer rather than focusing attention on the problem and its origin. Although we know that some diseases, such as cardiovascular disorders, are influenced by personal behavior (stress, diet, sedentary life, smoking), it is equally well known that personal behavior is itself influenced by social status, educational level, and peer pressure. A typical example is smoking, which today tends to be more widespread among the poorer classes and is gradually spreading in the less developed countries as the market shrinks in the wealthier countries (1 percent less every year in the northern hemisphere, 2 percent more every year in the southern hemisphere). As Minkler has stressed, historically, the principal blame for disease and accidents in the workplace has almost always been laid on workers rather than employers, who are more powerful and less vulnerable (35). The contemporary emphasis on personal health may accentuate this trend.

Another consequence is the attitude revealed by the idea that workers exposed to carcinogens in the workplace *must* learn not to smoke, in order to reduce their risks of cancer; the person working in constantly stressful conditions *must* learn to relax. In other words, responsibility for the health of workers in hazardous conditions is implicitly shifted from employer to employee; imposing healthy personal behavior is a cheaper and less demanding alternative for employers than are technical, organizational, and environmental solutions. Allegrante and Sloan conclude: "We do not mean to suggest that individuals have no responsibility whatsoever in disease causation; such an assertion would be false and irresponsible. However, blame for lung cancer, for example, cannot be assigned exclusively to an individual who [is] bombarded with persuasive messages from advertisers or who works with known carcinogens on a daily basis. . . . The use of behavior-change strategies must be balanced with enlightened practices designed to address organizational-level factors contributing to health risk" (34, pp. 315–316).

These reflections may be supplemented by other questions with ethical implications. Who decides on these strategies? And for whom? Who informs and who is informed? On the basis of what facts is policy formulated? This last question conjures up complex and contradictory issues that I shall mention in passing, including the relationship between notions and prejudice in scientific knowledge; the power of physicians (and of epidemiologists in particular) to determine what healthy behavior is; and, above all, the right of everyone to choose an individual "lifestyle."

The Risks and Benefits

Comparative evaluations of risks and benefits, in relation to the health of workers, have always started from an initial question: what levels of harmfulness and risk are acceptable? One result of research has been the gradual introduction of guidelines limiting the concentration of environmental hazards in the workplace, first for chemical substances and later for physical factors (radiation, noise, etc.) and, in certain cases, for organizational conditions (e.g., work rhythms). Indeed, the limits were originally defined with respect to the "maximum admissible concentration" (MAC), which set a maximum value that must never be exceeded; this measurement, however, was followed by the "threshold limit value" (TLV), which determines the mean concentration per shift, and by other indicators.

These guidelines proved useful both as an acknowledgment of a problem and as an effort at a solution. They were either introduced by law or, as in Italy, first adopted in labor contracts as a result of trade union efforts and then translated into legislation. This was the case in the 1960s for chemical workers' contracts, which adopted the values set by the American Conference of Governmental Industrial Hygienists. The MAC and TLV values were, however, determined based on factors that varied over time, including the risk factor investigated and the sophistication of research methods. Furthermore, for factors such as carcinogens, no "dosage" can be assessed as having no risk, which means that, logically, a threshold near zero should be mandated for such factors.

Over time these evaluations of risk factors have become the focus of bitter social clashes, especially when limits are constantly revised downward as researchers report harmful effects at concentrations previously considered acceptable. Still, the guidelines, by codifying tolerable risk levels, ensure continuity of production, which is seen as all-important for the economic health of the nation as a whole. Thus, the issue of guidelines for workplace hazards has given rise to numerous scientific and juridical controversies (e.g., 36). Workers may face times of dramatic difficulty when they have little power, when the state is disinclined to interfere, and when the actions of companies reflect the absence of rules and of respect for human life. On the other hand, when conditions change, workplace risks can diminish; in some cases, they may even become lower than those encountered off the job.

Besides the question of "acceptable risk," there is another question that is often neglected and may be expressed very simply: whose risk—and whose benefit? The ethical problem lies in the fact that, in the vast majority of cases, an asymmetry exists: one group incurs the risk while another reaps the benefit. We have already seen the problem expressed in the words of Leopardi (10); since his time, the question "Is it right?" has constantly been asked. For example, does the usefulness of the minerals extracted justify miners working in such hazardous and unhealthy conditions (37)?

The justification customarily invoked is that of a "superior interest," such as national defense or economic progress; but horrible misdeeds may be committed in its name. At the first International Congress of the History of Working and Environmental Prevention (Rome, 1998), researchers disclosed that, from 1947 to 1966, workers of the Navajo nation were routinely exposed to radiation in the mining and processing of uranium (38). The total lack of information about the risks of radiation given to the miners and grinders of uranium (risks known at that time), the obstacles to all controls, and the absence of any safeguards were at the time seen as justified by the value of uranium in U.S. military strategy. A long time later, representatives of the U.S. Department of Energy admitted that miners and grinders had been "unwitting and involuntary victims of human experiments, deliberately exposed in order to assess the effects of radiation on health." The final report of the inquiry acknowledged that "the uranium miners are the single group that was put most seriously at risk of harm, with inadequate disclosure and with often fatal consequences. The failure of the government and its researchers to adequately warn uranium miners, who were continually being studied, is difficult to comprehend; but the greater question is why, with the knowledge that they had, government agencies did not act to reduce risk in the mines in the first place" (38).

One of many possible explanations is that of the "reverse selection" of workers belonging to less protected ethnic groups, as discussed previously. At the same 1998 International Congress where the story of the Navaho uranium miners was presented, researchers reported the case of 1,126 Italian migrants who, from 1946 to 1966, uninformed and unprotected, worked in crocidolite (blue asbestos) mines in Australia (39). Subsequent epidemiological surveys showed that deaths due to mesothelioma, the cancer caused by asbestos, were higher among the Italians than among other workers, which suggests that the Italian workers were employed in the riskiest areas and activities.

I fear that, unless there are substantial improvements in the riskiest workplaces, researchers 10 or 20 years hence will be reporting the diseases of North African migrant farm laborers working in Italy, where they are the workers subjected to the heaviest toil. And I ask myself what possible justification there can be for cases like these in the light of the fundamental principles of ethics. In the words of the utilitarian principle asserted by Francis Hutcheson, "The best action is the one that produces the greatest happiness for the greatest number; the worst is the one that likewise produces suffering" (40). And again, in the principle of justice as stated by John Rawls: "Economic and social inequality must be for the greatest benefit of the less advantaged" (41).

CONFLICTS ON INFORMATION AND SCIENTIFIC RESEARCH

The knowledge of ourselves, which is intrinsically connected with human nature and aspirations, includes a profound mastery of our activities. Until comparatively recently, work knowledge consisted of little beyond a tradition in which apprentices acquired the secrets of a trade, literally hands-on, directly from experienced masters. The complexity of the modern workplace has extended the scope but also diminished the immediacy of this knowledge. That complexity will only increase as researchers in many fields—physiology and psychology, anthropology and ergonomics, biochemistry and biology, medicine and information science—continue their work-related studies.

The increasing quantity and complexity of information concerning jobs and workplaces underlines the worker's right to and desire for knowledge, especially crucial where its denial can increase the risk to workers of physical or psychological harm. Knowledge implies, first as humane impulse and then as legal regulation, a recognition of the worker's right to know all aspects of the job. With regard to health issues, this right includes (*a*) collection of data concerning the health and environmental consequences of productive activities for both individuals and communities and (*b*) availability of and access to these data for all those with a legitimate interest in them.

The primary source of work-related information is, of course, scientific research. Here, too, there is no lack of areas of conflict. The director of the U.S. National Institute for Occupational Safety and Health (NIOSH), Linda Rosenstock, has analyzed global threats deriving from political decisions and special interests (42); among political decisions she cites the actions of 104th Congress, which, in the Contract With America, reduced or abolished many educational, work, and health programs and cut public funding of research. She further reports that the two international organizations concerned with the protection of health, the World Health Organization and the International Labor Office, released technical reports on the asbestos industry that had been manipulated (43). The special interests cited by Rosenstock mainly included the industries that sponsor research designed (*a*) to demonstrate the absence of harmful effects caused by their products (the most glaring example being the tobacco industry), (*b*) to increase uncertainty with respect to harmfulness in order to avoid doing what is required in the light of already documented evidence, or (*c*) to suggest procedures that can serve to slow or block intervention.

Sometimes special interests—or social prejudices—foster "sins of omission" in the allocation of funds to research programs, or else distort evaluation of the subjects and the facts. For example, one scholarly article asserted that whenever female Jewish workers have a work-related accident they "become nervous, querulous, and introspective and complain of insomnia, dizziness, buzzing in the ears, and pain practically everywhere, which has no real location but originates in the brain" (44). Researchers of the conflict between reproductive function and health viewed the problem (as we shall see) almost exclusively as a function of women's work, neglecting the male factors involved in prenatal pathology. The conclusion reached by Rosenstock in her analysis was that "the scientific community must work together to defend the basic principles of scientific enquiry from such attempts to foster revisionist science" (42, p. 113). It might be added: the defense of those basic principles must proceed in the name of the critical importance of disinterested research, as embodied in the right of all to untainted scientific information.

A note by Vicente Navarro[1] summed up several of the difficulties involved in asserting this right. One is that workers must themselves initiate the request for information, when there are many brutal or subtle ways of preventing them from doing so. Another is that, in many cases, workers may not know they have any reason for requesting such information, as a particular occupational disease may not manifest itsel before an exposure of many years (as in, for example, cancer), or may be nonspecific (e.g., chronic bronchitis and emphysema), or may remain subclinical and insidious for years (e.g., the neuro-behavioral effects of lead). The right to know may also be denied on the basis of industrial secrecy, a form of self-protection acknowledged by law in all countries, which sometimes is used not as a rule for fairness in economic competition but to limit access to information by a company's own workers. Navarro added in his note that in the United States the Supreme Court has further protected this secrecy, asserting that inspections may not be performed without prior notification of the company, which allows the

[1] The note, "An International Study on Ethics and Values in Occupational Medicine," a personal communication dated March 1982, formed the introduction to a research project and was a stimulus to many of my present ideas.

latter to correct and conceal any unhealthy or dangerous conditions before the inspection is carried out.

But even where, as in most European countries, legislation guarantees workers the right to be informed, the corresponding requirements are hardly ever enforced—namely, the responsibility of the company (45) to provide not only standardized information (labels, lists of substances used, environmental and health data) but also such information as is immediately necessary for health and safety. In some countries, such as Italy, workers have established the right of access to outside professional assistance, in recognition of the fact that company-employed specialists can produce reports biased towards the interests of the company and against those of the workers. It may be added that, when scientific research (or evidence from the workers themselves) has revealed that certain substances or procedures in the workplace are harmful, companies have often attempted to conceal the facts or to encourage elusive interpretations in order to avoid compensating the workers affected or making changes to the company's production setup.

Many illuminating cases are described in the scientific literature. Two of the cases—exposure to radon in uranium mines and the possible carcinogenic effects of chlorophenoxyacetic weedkillers—have been described by O. Axelson (46). That of asbestos was thoroughly studied, including the use of archival research, by Lilienfeld and Engin (47). From a reconstruction of their knowledge of pneumoconiosis (accumulation of dust in the lungs) and of tumors caused by asbestos, it emerges that the two company doctors who identified the disease, Lanza and Gardner, were long prevented from publishing the results of their research. Research on the possible cancer-causing effects of asbestos was undertaken in 1936 on the basis of an agreement between the manufacturing companies and the Saranac Laboratory that stated, "The results obtained will be considered the property of those who are providing the research funds and who will determine whether, to what extent, and in what manner they shall be made public."

This statement has not the slightest justification in the name of industrial secrecy, which may be invoked only to forestall illegal competition and thus refers to products and processes, not to issues involving the health and safety of workers. Two ethical and juridical problems thus arise. The first is related to the fundamental ethical principle of science—freedom. And freedom of research necessarily includes the freedom to communicate knowledge. Without this freedom, a scientist is undeserving of the name, the "scientific community" ceases to exist, and the path of scientific progress itself is strewn with obstacles. The second problem may be expressed in the form of a question: how can it be right for companies to treat as private property information vital to persons exposed to hazards of disease or death, in the interest of avoiding paying insurance premiums or compensation or even of maintaining the unhealthy conditions?

On the other hand, even without special agreements (such as the one regarding asbestos, similar forms of which are often still used in the relations between industry and scientific research), this confiscation of vital information is still common practice. When, for instance, at Seveso, in northern Italy, a chemical reactor at the ICMESA factory exploded and released a thick dioxin-containing cloud into the surrounding area, the subsequent parliamentary inquiry revealed that knowledge of the danger was inversely proportional to exposure to risk. The management of the chemical reactor's owner, the Swiss-based multinational corporation Hoffman–La Roche, was fully aware of the danger. Indeed, the plant itself had been deliberately built on the Italian side of the natural barrier formed by the Alps, which retained the toxic cloud in the Po Valley in Italy. At Seveso, the technicians and managers possessed some scanty information, while the workers and the inhabitants of the area knew nothing, not even that the highly toxic substance called dioxin existed. On a much larger scale, there is an even more serious imbalance in relative knowledge between the northern and southern hemispheres of the world. Asbestos, for example, continues to be mined, produced, and used in many countries, with neither workers nor population aware of its harmfulness.

In ascertaining and transmitting health and safety information for the workplace, the most conflicted role may be that of the industrial physician. A corporate filter may influence even the normal doctor-patient relationship. What information concerning the worker must be given to the company, and what information concerning the company is the doctor authorized to give the worker? The ethical dilemmas and professional conflicts of this atypical figure in medicine are widely debated in bioethical and forensic medical literature. B. Walker wrote that, only too often, many industrial health professionals have taken the attitude that the company is always right, pointing out that economic interests can lead to a position of "unilateral loyalty." He concludes with this statement: "Unquestionably, the goal of a health company and the goal of health workers may collide, and when they do come into conflict, occupational health personnel must be aware of their ethical responsibility to the health of the workers and to the principles of occupational medicine" (25, p. 1844).

There have been fewer but nevertheless significant discussions of ethical conflicts for researchers, whether involved in biological or clinical experiments on toxicity or studying epidemiology in the field. Having established that a substance or process is harmful, whom do you inform of this, and how? Sometimes you keep silent so as not to get involved. Other times, in the uncertainty that characterizes much biological research, but more frequently epidemiological research, the temptation prevails to "protect" workers against dangers that have yet to be conclusively proven to exist. To what extent is this an alibi for a lack of confidence in the capacity of workers to understand and evaluate scientific data?

The concept of the "professional secret" can be valid, as when the disclosing of information concerning individual workers could be detrimental to them. But when a collective damage may arise out of the opposite situation—that is, from withholding information in the name of industrial secrecy that concerns harmful or hazardous activities—compulsory disclosure should apply as the ethical rule and should be considered as binding as are rules of secrecy for physicians and researchers. Bringing these two obligations together, article 105 of the Brazilian Code of Medical Ethics is extremely precise in prohibiting the disclosure "of confidential information obtained during the medical examination of the worker, even if the request is made by the company management or by institutions, unless silence would be detrimental to the health of the workers or of the community" (48).

CONFLICTS BETWEEN PRODUCTION AND ENVIRONMENT, WORKERS AND POPULATION

From the dawn of the Industrial Revolution until a few decades ago, only a handful of isolated and unheeded scientists and politicians warned of the dangers of environmental contamination and, more generally, of alterations in the biosphere. The prevailing opinion when evidence of environmental damage could no longer be ignored was that it was the inevitable price to be paid for progress. Indeed, for a long time, when the most serious diseases studied were those of microbial origin and researchers first hypothesized and then demonstrated that the transmission of infection occurred by direct contagion or through food, arthropods, air, and water, few suspected the existence of another kind of "contagion": the spread of pathogenic factors from the workplace to the outside environment. Only very recently have the agents of transmission been traced from factories to consumers, in products themselves (for instance, asbestos), and in the release of pollutants into the air, water, and soil (and from the latter into food, as in the case of pesticides), but also in such seemingly unrelated categories as energy consumption and the relationship between work and rest. And yet the effects of pollution have been known since ancient times. Ramazzini mentions them in his book, in the chapter on the diseases of chemists (2, p. 51). He describes a "violent dispute" between an inhabitant of Finale (Modena) and "a certain business man who owned a huge laboratory at Finale where he manufactured sublimate" that polluted the surrounding air, making it so damaging to the lungs that the parish records revealed a higher mortality in the area surrounding the laboratory. In the end, writes Ramazzini, "the jury sustained the manufacturer, and vitriol was found not guilty. Whether the legal expert judged correctly I shall leave to the judgment of the experts in natural science." It may be further postulated that the verdict was influenced by the different social positions of the two legal counsels: the local doctor acting as counsel for the villagers and the artillery commissioner for the Duke of Este acting for the merchant, and we may suspect that the clash between juridical and natural science was an uneven match between two powers of different strengths.

Awareness of industrial sources of contagion lagged behind that of diseases of microbial origin, despite the fact that microbial infection is due to invisible organisms (Mark Twain wrote that their invisibility was an ingenious and wicked idea of the Creator, who for thousands of years had prevented man from knowing of their existence and thus from dominating disease), while industrial hazards to health are often directly perceptible through the natural use of the senses. One reason for the comparative neglect of the role of industry in spreading disease could be that the advantages deriving from industrial progress were so great as to overshadow the damage. My evaluation is that, as in the discussion on risks and benefits, judgment may have been influenced by an asymmetry: those enjoying the advantages had a stronger voice than the person suffering the damage.

The environmental problem must also be evaluated on the basis of the ethical category of justice. The use of the word "contagion" is not simply metaphorical. Workers are usually the first to experience disease or damage when a new industrial production is introduced. These same workers are, as a result, often the guinea pigs in large-scale experiments designed to determine the patho-genic effects of chemical substances or physical factors—experiments carried out without the informed consent of the participants, while the products (and the pathogens) are distributed through the marketplace to the population.

Workers often suffer twice from these effects: at work and at home. Carl Talbot, with reference both to this phenomenon and to the locations of polluting factories, spoke of the existence of "class and race relations" that have led to "environmental injustice," in the sense that "some parts of the population shoulder a dispro-portionate burden of the negative effects of environmental degradation" (49). Talbot cites as an example the "environmental racism" suffered by the Irish immigrants to Manchester in the midnineteenth century, who were obliged to live in conditions of "filth, degeneration and squalor, in contempt of all conditions of cleanliness, ventilation and hygiene" (50). Another example is the recent analysis, sponsored by the United Church of Christ, of the location of toxic waste treatment industries in the United States (51, cited in 49), which reveals that race is the most significant variable in the geographic distribution of polluting industries, above all to the detriment of Hispanic-American communities. At the international level, geographic inequality can also be seen in the export by developed countries of toxic and harmful waste to poor countries (52; see also 53), with the country of origin sometimes paying monetary compensation, sometimes dumping the waste illegally. In many cases, "double standards" of occupational hygiene and environmental safety are adopted.

In reaction to these abuses, an awareness grew that human beings have a right to work and live in a healthy environment. The first voices arguing on behalf of this right began to be heard in the factories as early as the eighteenth century; in recent decades, this argument has expanded to embrace the destiny of all life on our "only planet." One may wonder, however, why the two most important environmental movements of the past few decades—the movements championing workers' health and the protection of the natural environment—have been so distant from each other, sometimes clashing bitterly. According to Talbot, this is because "capitalism succeeded in promoting the belief that the industrial control regulations aimed at protecting the environment led to loss of jobs; it thus succeeded in creating the myth of 'work versus environment,' which is translated into 'workers versus environmentalists,' which creates deep divisions between labor movements and environmental movements" (49, p. 99).

However, the estrangement of the two movements cannot be the only cause of slow progress in controlling industrial pollution. To this must be added scientific ignorance, inertia, the vacillation of institutions, and the lack of suitable laws, as well as the deafness of members of the two movements to each other's ideas. Above all, we must remember that control of potential industrial pollution can only be instituted efficiently at the planning stage of industrial operations, by analyzing future impact. If this is not done, the costs become unsustainable—in terms of health, the environment, and the economy, but also in terms of social strife and personal hardship, as when conflicts arise within families and communities. In many of the examples cited, clashes occurred between workers and their families. The ethical problem in conflicts between the legitimate interests of workers and of populations can only rarely be solved after the fact, as this would mean sacrificing either the one or the other. The problem is that such externalities are not taken into account in economic calculations, and intangible goods such as the physical integrity of workers and the safeguarding of the environment are assessed as having zero value.

However, that these costs do exist means that health and safety, considerations that are otherwise liable to be compromised, should be included from the very beginning of the design and estimation phase in industrial planning for maximum advantage at the production and consumption stages. Of course, the proponents of health and safety restrictions must also take into account the fact that, in the absence of production, unemployment and poverty lead to disease and environmental degradation. The chances of this design-and-forecast approach coming into common use would be increased by a rapprochement of the two movements, which have hitherto been so combative. According to Epelman, this requires overcoming the reciprocal prejudices: "On the one hand, workers often think that the environmental movement, in its action against pollution, threatens the source of their jobs. For their part, environmentalists consider that the trade union movement is interested only in struggling for economic claims" (54). I do not think that these are simply prejudices: in many instances, they are post hoc judgments arrived at, on both sides, from experience. The need is clear, however, for an approach based on a convergence of interests, that is, on the need to devise ways to control pollution while maintaining the economic health of workers and communities.

I have spoken so far of the conflicts and ethical problems in many countries. Together with these, three additional complex issues are emerging, which I shall outline only briefly. The first is that of *the world space*. Faced with rules and movements intended to regulate the impact of industrial activity on health and the environment in the developed countries, multinational corporations (as well as some smaller companies) are increasingly transferring their operations to poor countries. The exportations include both banned products, such as asbestos and coloring agents known to cause cancer, and toxic wastes produced by the factories. Thus, two regulatory systems have been set up, corresponding to two different estimations of the value of human work, life, and the environment (55): literally a moral double standard. For some time now, the WHO and IARC (the International Cancer Research Agency) have been focusing attention on this issue, although no significant reversal of the trend has occurred so far.

The second issue is *generational time,* that is, the effects of our actions on future generations and on the global equilibrium of the biosphere. H. Jonas has pointed out the difficulty of equating the question of rights raised by this problem to other existing rights. He wrote that the precept of "once certain rights of others have been established, it follows that I have the duty to respect them and, if possible, to promote them" does not work in this case: indeed, "the nonexistent cannot advance any claim and cannot even suffer a violation of its rights" (56, p. 49). He added, however, that this ethical problem must be tackled just the same, as "a metaphysical responsibility in its own right, since man has become a danger not only to himself but also to the entire biosphere." So, in grappling with this question of the future fate of the earth, "man's interest coincides in the loftiest sense with the rest of life, as it is his cosmic home." It is thus possible to apply the guiding concept of "duty towards man" without slipping into reductive anthropocentrism (56, p. 175). However, we can see how remote these ideas are from the method and substance of politics in its everyday practice. Democracy must also be a vehicle of expression for those who cannot express themselves, that is, for those yet to be born, who vastly outnumber the human beings actually alive today, and for the other species that have evolved and coexist with us.

The third issue involves *the duty to act in conditions of scientific uncertainty*. In many cases, the health and environmental consequences of industrial operations are still unknown. In others, however, despite the uncertainty about what form the damage will take, one thing is certain: unless prompt action is taken, any reparative action will be too late and the resultant damage irreversible. The best-known examples are those of global-scale climatic changes due to carbon dioxide emissions and the thinning of the ozone shield layer; but there are also cases related to carcinogens in the workplace and the environment. The medical principle *in dubium abstine,* aimed at avoiding action possibly harmful to the patient in case of doubt, should be applied as an ethical principle in both actions and omissions that might cause irreversible collective damage. The burden of proof of nontoxicity ought in this case to replace the burden of proof of damage, according to the "precaution principle."

CONFLICTS AMONG WORKERS

Conflicts of bioethical significance may arise among workers when, for example, a worker is affected by mental disease, contagious physical disease, or psycho-sensory disability, or adopts behavior potentially harmful to others. This may happen in various ways: direct transmission, by "contagion" of the unhealthy habits to other workers (including, in the case of some forms of drug addiction, initiation of those workers into use of the drug); reduce collaboration in working activities; or increased likelihood of accidents. These are not new issues. In recent years there has been debate over additional bioethical questions raised by the presence in the workplace of HIV-positive subjects, the demonstration of the pathogenic effects of "passive smoking," and the use of such true or alleged risk indicators as genetic testing.

We must not forget that these conflicts can develop complex moral dimensions. For example, everyone has the right to work, the right not to be discriminated against on the grounds of biology or pathology. Indeed, this right takes on special significance when the work itself can have a supporting or therapeutic function, in cases of, for example, mental illness or physical impairment or drug addiction. Experience has shown—and this is one of the most encouraging ethical developments of the past few decades—that inclusion in the world of work can radically improve these conditions. And in such cases, exclusion or segregation may only aggravate the problem. On the other hand, "normal" or "healthy" workers have the right not to suffer damage, not to be exposed to additional hazards because of the health status or the behavior of other workers. Furthermore, even if only in rare cases, these conditions or behaviors can represent a danger to persons other than co-workers—for example, to passengers in trains and aircraft. In practice, the objective must be to balance solidarity with those who suffer, and acceptance and support of the "abnormal," against the need for safety and security for all.

This type of conflict cannot be ignored. In some cases it is indeed necessary to take precautionary measures against workers that are actually dangerous and even to remove them from the workplace. On most occasions, however, the problem is aggravated by prejudices that tend to exaggerate the risk, and even to invent it when there is none, as happens in the majority of cases concerning workers with mental disorders, drug addictions, or HIV. The stigmatization of certain diseases and certain behaviors can blind co-workers to objective facts, blindness aggravated by an information gap or by viewpoints in which some fears are amplified and others repressed. It is typical in the debate concerning risks and conflicts among workers (or between workers and management) that, thanks to the protests of working women, sexual violence and harassment—probably the most widespread category of workplace conflict—have only recently been brought to the surface. On the other hand, the linking of the concept of violence with that of harassment for the purpose of combating both, in the name of the integrity and autonomy of women's bodies and minds, represents a significant ethical step forward in relations between the sexes.

In all fields, whenever conflicts among workers (or between male and female workers) have been viewed objectively, solidarity has turned out to be reconcilable with safety. Even in cases of seemingly irreconcilable conflict, it has been possible to reduce the distance between the antagonists. Exemplary experiments have been conducted, for example, in integrating persons with physical and psycho-sensory disability, mentally illness, drug addiction, or HIV into the workplace. In the latter case, company health services have made positive contributions whenever occupational health and safety programs have adequately supported their actions (57). Several factors have proven most important for facilitating the integration of such workers: first and foremost, the sense of solidarity, which, given sympathetic support, has always existed among workers; second, the open-minded attitude of many entrepreneurs; and third, the laws prohibiting workplace discrimination on biopathological grounds. One of the more significant examples of the latter is the Italian AIDS legislation, which prohibits HIV testing by companies and bans the practice of excluding workers from jobs on the basis of HIV status, except in a very small number of occupations in which it would actually represent a hazard for other workers or for the general public.

One category of conflict among workers that cannot be ignored, and which has to date shown only minimal improvement, is that of relations between native-born and immigrant workers. Trade union organizations have sometimes taken action to protect immigrant workers, although not always with the same degree of commitment as for other workers. The fact remains that immigrant workers are almost always given the most fatiguing and harmful jobs, are paid less than native-born workers, enjoy little health and social security protection, live in unhealthy or precarious accommodations, and run the risk of being fired or even expelled from the country. These facts hold true both for western European countries and for the United States. Italy is the only one of these countries to have had two opposite experiences, in the nineteenth and twentieth centuries: first, mass emigration of more than 25 million Italians; now, immigration of workers from Africa, the Middle East, Asia, and Latin America. Italians ought, therefore, to display a greater sensitivity than other nationalities. In fact, Italians are as prone to ethnic or geographic stereotyping as are any of the European or American citizens.

CONFLICT BETWEEN WORK AND REPRODUCTIVE HEALTH AND THE RIGHTS OF THE NEWBORN

I have already cited the Encyclical of John XXIII, *Pacem in terris* (14), as one of the basic documents of a modern ethics of labor relations, without discussing one provision that establishes a right specific to women: "the right to working conditions compatible with their needs and their duties as wives and mothers."

As we know, the Industrial Revolution for a long time ignored even the most elementary requirements of working women. In the 1st International Congress on Occupational Diseases, held in Milan in 1906, Francesco Pestalozza summed up the consequences as follows: "Gynecological diseases are much more frequent in the industrial regions than in the non-industrial districts; with increasing women's employment in the factories and fields, there is an increase in the number of miscarriages, premature births, and infant mortality; mortality is higher in the children of poor mothers working in the factories than in poor non-working mothers; morbidity and mortality in newborns and unweaned children are extremely high in children born to and suckled by undernourished mothers intoxicated by chronic overwork and occupational poisons" (58).

This first phase was followed by a second, more enlightened phase, characterized by the development of mother-child assistance and disease prevention and, above all, by the reduction of both the physical demands and working hours of working women (although the "double job" done by women, inside and outside the home, was but little reduced). The results could be seen in the drastic reduction of the phenomena reported by Pestalozza, as well as in a large body of research and testimonies. One of the most moving (and authentically Kafkaesque) testimonies is to be found in Franz Kafka's diaries, in which he tells of his impressions of factory life when he had the job of "labor inspector" (59). This positive phase subsequently merged into a third phase, which I have analyzed elsewhere—that of transforming protection of women into an obstacle to their entry into and career in the workplace (60). One of the reasons—or pretexts—for this is protection of the health of the unborn child, on the grounds that the child's health could be threatened by the mother's working environment.

This is the meaning of John XXIII's phrase, which, in reducing the relationship between working and parenthood to the simple duties of "wives and mothers" without mentioning husbands and fathers, reaffirms the Catholic Church's traditional position on working women. That traditional position mirrors the one-sidedness of scientific research in this field: "Indeed, all research carried out on human reproductive hazards has analyzed the effects of women's exposure to potentially harmful substances; very little is known about the consequences of male exposure" (18, p. 1850). Yes, there are risks that arise in the last few months of pregnancy for mothers performing tiring, heavy work (though this now occurs primarily in the less developed countries; the developed countries generally provide ample protection against overwork for mothers in later stages of pregnancy). But the genetic or toxic hazards that can come into play at conception can originate in either parent.

This one-sidedness (61) has begun to give way to more evenhanded research methods. However, from the ethical point of view, attention is still entirely focused on the conflict between the woman's right to work and the rights of the unborn child (e.g., 62). As a result, many U.S. industries have adopted "maternity protection" policies, in which women of childbearing age are advised to transfer to "healthy duties"; whenever the transfer is found to be impossible, many are simply fired. The attractive idea that, in so doing, "priority is given to the protection of the future generations" does not stand up to scientific scrutiny, for three reasons.

First, research into the effects of some toxic substances (such as lead) on reproductive health has shown that exposure is equally dangerous for young men and women (63). Convincing scientific evidence also exists to show that the father's exposure to radiation is associated with leukemia in future children, but no one has ever suggested excluding men from work involving this hazard in order to protect any children they might have. The second reason is that women are usually not given a choice between one job and another but, rather, between working and being unemployed, a condition in which the risks for the unborn child are much greater. Finally, the third reason (already mentioned) is that resolving ethical and practical conflicts by moving "more susceptible" subjects away from workplace hazards, whether male or female, young or old, strong or weak, is not only discrimination but also an obstacle to instituting preventive measures for those concerned and for everyone else. Indeed, exactly the same factors that affect "susceptible" workers also affect workers considered "normal," albeit to a lesser degree. In absolute figures and expressed as years of life lost, the damage is probably greater among the latter group.

Company policies can also ban women from the workplace on the grounds of "fetal protection" policies, sometimes using barbaric methods. For example, the management of the American Cyanamid Company, a U.S. chemical giant, ordered that women who were not sterile or willing to be sterilized must be excluded from departments exposed to lead hazard, offering the sterilization operation free and, in the case of refusal, transferring the women to another job (64, 65). However, only seven of the 30 women to be excluded were actually given another job; many were dismissed, and five chose "voluntary" sterilization in order to keep their jobs. The painful choice—job or motherhood—was apparently made in each case of the woman's free will, but was actually made by the company in its refusal to modify the hazardous conditions of the production cycle. Other methods, arguably even more barbaric, have been reported in less developed countries. In a Sri Lanka firm, for example, women of childbearing age were required to undergo a compulsory pregnancy test; those found to be pregnant were given the opportunity—but were actually required—to undergo an abortive curettage (66).

Nevertheless, alternatives exist between more or less compulsory sterilization or abortion and the loss of a job. The principal alternative is effective environmental preventive measures for all. The other solutions have both advantages and drawbacks. In Italy and in other developed countries, legislation prescribes pregnancy leave (with the employer prohibited from dismissing the expectant mother) during the final months of pregnancy and the first few months after childbirth. But it is now known that the most serious damage occurs during the early stages of pregnancy, often before pregnancy is detected. The legislation thus needs to be updated. And, given that harm to the unborn child may be due not only to maternal but also to paternal causes, it seems unlikely that harm can be avoided through legislative measures and through scrutiny of, for example, the sexual behavior inside and outside marriage of all the male workers exposed to workplace hazards. In any case, all those called upon to resolve such a difficult conflict—the legislator, the trade union representatives, and the worker, male or female—must have access to objective scientific information and must be allowed to decide on the basis of facts, not prejudice, in complete freedom and according to his or her own lights.

THE SETTLEMENT OF CONFLICTS

Conflicts can often arise from a power and information imbalance. When an employer's power dominates a conflict with employees, health and dignity can suffer, sometimes to the extent of reducing the length and quality of life of employees. Conflict between profit and the worker's integrity and dignity can become a question of professional ethics. A survey of U.S. industrial physicians on their ethical beliefs revealed how difficult reconciling such moral dilemmas can be, especially for those caught in the middle (67). This dilemma, for physicians who see themselves as having to choose between the welfare of the individual worker and corporate profit, is as unfair as it is unnecessary. A company's choosing to recognize the importance of the health and welfare of its workers and act accordingly is not necessarily incompatible with profit. Indeed, doing so has often stimulated productive transformations, in materials, processes, work organization, and products, and guaranteed both economic progress and social justice.

The various conflicts I have examined here are not likely just to disappear. In many cases, however, they may be avoided, or the extent and seriousness of their effects may be diminished. The history of conflicts between workers and employers shows that such disputes are less dramatic when a greater balance of power exists between the two contenders. Conflicts over information, for example, have often been resolved through guarantees of access to information pertinent to the health of workers and guarantees of the confidentiality of personal data about individual workers. Conflicts between workers and population and between production and environment have not even arisen where planners have made prior assessments of the health and environmental impacts of new plants. The conflicts between "dangerous" and "normal" workers are reduced to a handful of cases when the extent of a hazard is evaluated on the basis of objective data rather than prejudices. When the spirit of integration gains the upper hand over victim-blaming and segregation, workers grow in understanding and in appreciation for the role of ethics in personal relations.

Of course, these experiences cannot always resolve conflicts involving values and interests that are in some cases incompatible, nor can they always serve as a theoretical guide to making difficult and contradictory choices. However, the more bioethical concepts are applied in the course of everyday life, the more trusted these concepts will become as a point of reference for workers, both male and female—and, indeed, for everybody.

REFERENCES

1. Rossi, G. Si invoca l'etica quando è in crisi il diritto. *Corriere della Sera,* May 26, 1987.
2. Ramazzini, B. *De Morbis Artificum Diatriba.* Mutinae, 1700 (*Diseases of Workers,* New York Academy of Medicine, Hafner, New York, 1964).
3. Hume, D. Trattato sulla natura umana. In *Opere filosofiche,* vol. 1, p. 387. Laterza, Rome, 1999.
4. Louden, R. B. Virtue ethics. In *Encyclopedia of Applied Ethics,* edited by R. Chadwick, vol. 4, p. 491. Academic Press, San Diego, 1998.
5. Smith, A. *Ricerca sopra la natura e le cause della ricchezza delle nazioni (An Enquiry into the Nature and Causes of the Wealth of Nations),* p. 120. Newton, Rome, 1995.
6. Rothschild, E. Social security and laissez faire in eighteenth century political economy. *Popul. Dev. Rev.* 21(4): 712–717, 1995.
7. Malthus, T. R. An essay on the principle of population. In *The Works of T. R. Malthus,* edited by E. A. Wrigley and D. Souden, vol. 1. William Pickering, London, 1986.
8. Friedman, M. The responsibility of business is to make profit. *New York Time Magazine,* September 13, 1970, p. 32.
9. Lee, P. W. Some ethical problems of hazardous substances in the working environment. *Br. J. Indust. Med* 34: 274–280, 1977.
10. Leopardi, G. *Zibaldone,* nn. 1172–1173, p. 272. Newton, Rome, 1997.
11. Marx, K. *Il Capitale: Critica dell'economia politica,* vol. 1. Edizioni Rinascita, Rome, 1962.
12. Lafargue, P. *Il diritto alla pigrizia,* p. 96. Ed. Forum, Milan, 1968.
13. Smith, A. *Teoria dei sentimenti morali (The Theory of Moral Sentiments).* Rizzoli, Milan, 1995.
14. Pope John XXIII. *Pacem in terris.* Vatican City, April 11, 1963.
15. Pan-American Health Organization. *Declaration on Workers' Health.* Washington, D.C., February 6, 1992.
16. International Commission on Occupational Health. *International Code of Ethics for Occupational Health Progessionals.* 1992.
17. Kant, I. Idee per una storia universals dal punto di vista cosmopolitico. In *Scritti di storia, politica e diritto,* p. 34. Laterza, Rome, 1995.
18. Murray, T. H. Occupational safety and health: Testing of the employees. In *Encyclopedia of Bioethics,* edited by W. T. Reich, vol. 5. Simon & Schuster, New York, 1995.
19. Murray, T. H. Warning: Screening workers for genetic risk. *Hasting Centers Rep.* 13(1): 5–8, 1983.
20. Office of Technology Assessment, U.S. Congress. *The Role of Gene Testing in the Prevention of Occupational Diseases.* Washington, D.C., 1983.
21. Cummins, M. *Human Heredity: Principles and Issues,* p. 406. West Publishing, St. Paul, Minn., 1988.

22. Nespor, S., Santosuosso, A., and Satolli, R. *Vita, morte e miracoli,* pp. 97–112. Feltrinelli, Milan, 1992.
23. Rodotà, S. Test genetici per lavorare. *La Repubblica,* July 18, 1992.
24. Harris, J. Le biotecnologie nel 2000: Wonderwoman e Superman. *Bioetica* 1: 32, 1992.
25. Walker, B., Jr. Occupational safety and health: Occupational health care providers. In *Encyclopedia of Bioethics,* edited by W. T. Reich, vol. 4. Simon & Schuster, New York, 1995.
26. White House. *Executive Order: To Prohibit Discrimination in Federal Employment Based on Genetic Information.* Washington, D.C., February 8, 2000.
27. Ritter, G. *Storia dello stato sociale,* pp. 61–85. Laterza, Bari, 1996.
28. Righi, M. L. Le lotte per l'ambiente di lavoro dal dopoguerra ad oggi. *Studi Storici* 2/3: 619–652, 1992.
29. Berlinguer, G. *La salute nelle fabbriche,* expanded ed. De Donato, Bari, 1977 [1969].
30. Carnevale, F., and Moriani, G. Lavoro e lotte per la salute nel secondo dopoguerra. In *Storia della salute dei lavoratori,* pp. 131–194. Cortina, Verona, 1986.
31. Levenstein, C. Occupational safety and health: Ethical issues. In *Encyclopedia of Bioethics,* edited by W. T. Reich, vol. 4, p. 1842. Simon & Schuster, New York, 1995.
32. Berlinguer, G. Etica della prevenzione. In *Etica della salute,* 2d ed., pp. 95–106. EST, Milan, 1997.
33. Menlowe, M. A. Safety Laws. In *Encyclopedia of Applied Ethics,* edited by R. Chadwick, vol. 4, pp. 1–7. Academic Press, San Diego, 1998.
34. Allegrante, J. P., and Sloan, R. P. Ethical dilemmas in workplace health promotion. *Prev. Med* 15: 313–320, 1986.
35. Minkler, M. Ethical issues in community organization. *Health Educ. Monogr.* 6: 198–201, 1978.
36. Curran, W. J., Hyg, S. M., and Boden, L. I. Occupational health values in the Supreme Court: Cost-benefit analysis. *Am. J. Public Health* 71(11): 1264–1265, 1981.
37. Lee, W. R. Some ethical problems of hazardous substances in the working environment. *Br. J. Occup. Med.* 34: 274–280, 1977.
38. Moure-Eraso, R. Environmental impact of uranium mining in Navajo Nation 1947–1976: A case of human experimentation. In *Contributions to the History of Occupational and Environmental Prevention,* pp. 255–262. Elsevier, Amsterdam, 1999.
39. Merler, E., and Ercolanelli, M. On 1126 Italian migrants who worked at the crocidolite mine of Wittenoom Gorge between 1946 and 1966. In *Contributions to the History of Occupational and Environmental Prevention,* pp. 277–304. Elsevier, Amsterdam, 1999.
40. Hutcheson, F. Ricerca sulle idee di bellezza e di virtù. In *Gli illuministi inglesi,* edited by E. Lecaldano, p. 163. Loescher, Turin, 1985.
41. Rawls, J. *Una teoria della giustizia,* p. 225. Feltrinelli, Milan, 1993.
42. Rosenstock, L. Global threats to science: Policy, politics, and special interest. In *Contributions to the History of Occupational and Environmental Prevention,* pp. 111–113. Elsevier, Amsterdam, 1999.
43. Castleman, B. I., and Lemen, R. A. The manipulation of international scientific organizations (editorial). *Int. J. Occup. Environ. Health* 4(1): 53–55, 1998.
44. Dembe, A. E. The medical detection of simulated occupational injuries: A historical and social analysis. *Int. J. Health Serv.* 28: 233, 1998.

45. Walters, D. Health and safety in a changing Europe. *Int. J. Health Serv.* 28(2): 305–333, 1998.
46. Axelson, O. Etica, politica e interpretazione dell'evidenza scientifica dei rischi per la salute dovuti a esposizioni ambientali e professionali. *Epidemiologia e prevenzione* 42: 8–11, 1990.
47. Lilienfeld, D. E., and Engin, M. S. The silence: The asbestos industry and early occupational research: A case study. *Am. J. Public Health* 81(6): 791–800, 1991.
48. Pereira Dias, H. Bioethics: Implications for medical practice and deontological and legal standards in Brazil. In *Bioethics: Issue and Perspectives,* edited by S. Scholle Connor and H. L. Fuenzalida-Puelma, p. 138. Pan-American Health Organization, New York, 1990.
49. Talbot, C. Environmental justice. In *Encyclopedia of Applied Ethics,* edited by R. Chadwick, vol. 2, pp. 93–105. Academic Press, San Diego, 1998.
50. Engels, F. *La situazione della classe operaia in Inghilterra,* pp. 72–100. Edizioni Rinascita, Rome, 1955.
51. *Toxic Wastes and Race in the USA.* Public Data Access, New York, 1987.
52. Castleman, B. Global corporate policies and international 'double standards' in occupational and environmental health (editorial). *Int. J. Occup. Environ. Health* 5(1): 61–64, 1999.
53. Shrader-Frechette, A. Hazardous and toxic substances. In *Encyclopedia of Applied Ethics,* edited by R. Chadwick, vol. 4, pp. 525–532. Academic Press, San Diego, 1998.
54. Epelman, M. Sindicalismo y medio ambiente en Argentina. Unpublished paper. January 1992.
55. Comba, P. Il rischio ambientale e la salvaguardia della vita umana: aspetti etici. *Protestantesimo* 46(4): 287–300, 1991.
56. Jonas, H. *Il principio responsabilità: Un 'etica per la civiltà tecnologica.* Einaudi, Turin, 1990.
57. London, L. AIDS control and the workplace: The role of occupational health services in South Africa. *Int. J. Health Serv.* 28(3): 575–591, 1998.
58. Pestalozza, F. Il lavoro delle donne e la protezione della maternità. In *Atti del primo Congresso internazionale per le malattie del lavoro,* June 14, 1906, pp. 519–525. Reggiani, Milan, 1906.
59. Kafka, F. *Confessioni e diari,* pp. 322–323. Mondadori, Milan, 1972.
60. Berlinguer, G. Lavoro e salute riproduttiva: Traiettoria di un secolo. *Recenti progressi in medicina* 88(1): 470–478, 1997.
61. Figà Talamanca, I. *I tossici ambientali e riproduttivi e la riproduzione umana.* Piccin, Padua, 1994.
62. Lavine, M. Ethical and policy problems. *Environment* 24(5): 26–38, 1982.
63. Becker, M. E. Can employers exclude woman to protect children? *JAMA* 246(16): 2113–2117, 1990.
64. Hricko, A. Social policy consideration of occupational health standards: The example of lead and reproductive effects. *Prev. Med.* 7: 394–406, 1978.
65. Curran, J. Danger for pregnant women in the work place. *N. Engl. J. Med.,* January 17, 1985, pp. 164–165.
66. Figà Talamanca, I. Zone industriali libere e adolescenti sfruttate. *Salute umana* 107, 1990.
67. Brandt -Rauf, P. W. Ethical conflict in the practice of occupational medicine. *Br. J. Indust. Med.* 46: 63–66, 1989.

CHAPTER 4

The Human Body:
From Slavery to the Biomarket

THE MULTIDIMENSIONAL ENHANCEMENT
OF THE BODY

The conflicts of interest and value discussed in the preceding chapter refer to working relations as they now exist, between free moral subjects who are formally and legally autonomous. This was not always the case. For a very long time, during the age of slavery, labor was regulated through domination by the few and subjugation of many who were considered to have practically no rights at all.

To restrict the analysis of the relationship between scientific knowledge, material life, and ethical tendencies to free subjects living in the present age seems somewhat limiting. Even though the term "bioethics" was coined only 30 years ago, the concept is as old as the history of ideas and behaviors regarding birth, reproduction, work, disease, treatment, experimentation, and death. Historians tell us, for example, that, in eighteenth-century England the right to receive food and lodging from charitable institutions often implied a moral duty on the part of the beneficiaries (for whom the requirement represented a servitude or an implicit obligation) to make their bodies available for medical experimentation (1). We know from researchers who have traced back the origins of "informed consent" that, until the end of the eighteenth century, the century of *liberté*, "it was common practice to carry out research on slaves and servants without the subjects' knowledge or consent" (2). We know from the history of philosophy that Plato, at the time when Hippocrates was laying the foundations of scientific medicine and the physician's duty towards the patients, considered it normal and just to have two different categories of sick people—free men and slaves. The free man was well cared for and kept fully informed by free physicians about the prescribed treatment; the slave was hastily examined by a slave physician, who told the patient nothing and behaved like an "arrogant despot" (3).

A diachronic perspective may enhance our understanding of a bioethics that is based on the past as well as the present and future. For many problems this outlook is compulsory, as we live in a world in which, side by side with extraordinary innovations, we often encounter leftovers from and returns to earlier behaviors. However, this mix of past and present can represent an analytical advantage, as it allows us to make comparisons from which to draw useful conclusions. On the basis of these thoughts, the idea came to me to develop several observations on the reality and the culture of the human body over the past few decades.

It seems to me that the greatest novelty of the present day resides in the fact that never before has the human body been so widely (although not universally) secularized, respected, enhanced, and appreciated. The only comparison in western culture would appear to be in the attitude expressed in ancient Greece (although only regarding *free* men of *male* gender); but the conditions, means, values, and results are in actual fact anything but comparable.

As a case history and positive analysis of the present-day glorification of the human body, I refer, in a brief, nonsystematic, and incomplete list, to the following phenomena:

1. Recognition of the inviolability of the person, going well beyond the sphere of the original interpretations of *habeas corpus* (4)
2. The superseding of the claim (and of the acceptance) of women's biological inferiority (5)
3. Liberation and control of sexuality and reproduction, phenomena of great importance in the assertion of women's rights
4. A considerable lengthening of the average lifetime, now probably approaching the limits of the species, and the pursuit of a higher quality of life
5. The possibility of treating many "incurable" diseases and of preventing many "fatal" illnesses
6. Introduction of methods to correct and compensate for many physical, sensory, and mental disabilities, both prior to and after birth
7. Recognition of the right to health and safety as a fundamental right of the human being, and the confirmation—in view of the experience gained in numerous countries—that this can be achieved in practice
8. Enhanced respect for workers' bodies and their health and safety
9. The transition, in the case of accidents and diseases, from compensation related to working and earning capacity to compensation for "biological damage"
10. The widespread practice of physical exercise and sport, interpreted as physical freedom and the pursuit of "fitness" and improvement
11. Emergence of the view of patients as moral subjects no longer subordinated to the authority or paternalism of the physician
12. The possibility of removing, modifying, conserving, transferring, and using separate parts of the human body, to the benefit of others—blood; bone marrow; organs removed from corpses; male and female gametes from living donors—representing the success of biomedicine, often life-saving advantages for many persons, and actions that push forwards the frontiers of human solidarity.

Many other items could easily be added to this list. One could even challenge the list, by rejecting the idea that the phenomena described have an intrinsic positive moral content, or by emphasizing the limits and the distortions encountered in practical applications. I have already tried to answer some of the general objections based on other moral principles—for instance, objections regarding the liberating value of regulating births and the survival of the disabled. I cannot but agree with the objections concerning the limits and distortions likely to be encountered. Indeed, I confess that I intended to oppose to each positive item on the list another, negative item based on facts that contradict its claims. I did not do so because I thought I might already have been too ambitious and pedantic in compiling the first list. Furthermore, before analyzing the specifics of each item's limits and distortions, I would have had to precede each item with an acknowledgment of their collective inadequacy—namely, that access to all these benefits is selective and unjust, facts difficult to justify in moral terms. Finally, I refrained from compiling the second list because the central discussion in this chapter is not meant to be a detailed analysis of the pros and cons that today surround, involve, and shape the body of the present-day human being. The issue I wish to develop is the clash between the multidimensional enhancement of the status of the human body and the parallel growth of another phenomenon that is different—indeed, opposite—in nature: never before, except when slavery was rife, has the human body been so widely treated as mere commodity.

THE TRANSFORMATION OF BODY
TO COMMODITY

Several aspects of this commodification of the body are obvious to all and have even been mythologized as urban legend. The French M.P. Leon Schwartzenberg contributed to the irresponsible birth and spread of one such legend when, several years ago, he denounced in the European Parliament the alleged disappearance in Italy of three thousand children, adoptees from Brazil, insinuating that they had been used as a source of human organs (6). Thorough investigations proved the rumor was groundless. Other factual accounts of the "human market" appear from time to time in the news, based on single episodes or decisions that arouse comment—such as that of the European Patent Office to issue a patent for the production of embryos, including those of the human species. Between one legend and the next, and after each episode and decision, all public interest and concern subsides, to be replaced by silence and indifference. There is a lack of constant comprehensive information, and it is thus difficult to identify the connection between the facts and the policies and decisions that, in my opinion, converge in a definite tendency to adapt to the dictates of the world market.

The documentary and analytical deficit is probably related to the fact that the role now played by the market has been forgotten or underestimated in the bioethical debate. The subjects considered deserving of bioethical reflection are

men and women, human gametes and embryos, living species and their environments, medical and biological science and associated professions, public institutions, civil and criminal legislation, moral behaviors and trends. The market is
almost always excluded from such deliberations or considered to be of marginal
importance.

And yet the market has an increasing impact on the relationship between science
and material life, on principles and attitudes, on legislation and ideas. In discussing
the right to health in the modern state, for example, Dorothy Porter envisaged the
possibility during this century of the market replacing the state in the regulation of
health care (7). Although avoidable, this is actually what is happening: the market
is gaining the upper hand over moral issues in the field of health and is co-opting
those decisions, that throughout the twentieth century, were often made democrat-
ically and in the common interest. The diseases of the human body have become a
source of profit, and its image (particularly that of the female body) is used as a
vehicle to sell all kinds of commodities. Even more striking is a new phenomenon:
many human organs are now offered on the open market as "spare parts." This
most literal commodification of humans is linked to the possibility, previously
unavailable, of using separate parts of the body to treat diseases, to combat
sterility, to replace organs or damaged tissues. The irony is that the science that
pioneered the beneficial use of these "materials" at the same time opened the way
to their use as commodities.

Surprised and indignant at the emergence of this trend, several years ago a
Brazilian colleague, Volnei Garrafa, and I endeavored to set it in a comprehensible
framework. We drew up a "catalogue" of parts of the human body and compiled a
list of nations in which they were bought and sold, in order to highlight the
practical and ethical differences among the various human commodities (renew-
able and nonrenewable ones, for example) and to discuss the practical, scientific,
and ethical consequences (8; see also 9, the second edition of the book). Even more
than by the actual facts, we were surprised by the numerous voices of physicians,
jurists, and philosophers raised in favor of the more or less legal forms of this
market; that is, the substantial presence of a "justificatory bioethics." I could add,
irreverently and paradoxically, that (in this field as in others) justification is based
on the extension of the Hegelian principle according to which all that is real is
rational and, further, what is real must also be considered ethical. In practice, justificatory bioethics strives to legitimize the purchase, sale, hiring, and lending of the
human body. If this ethics were to prevail, the market would no longer have any
bounds and the human body would become "the final commodity"—with the consent of the medical profession, the permission of law, and the approval of philosophy.

ANALOGIES WITH SLAVERY

The book by Garrafa and myself extensively describes and comments on the
opinions expressed both for and against this "biomarketing." Before presenting

my comparison of the biomarket and slavery, I shall merely summarize one of the arguments used in support of this market: the analogies with other forms of "human commerce." If, biomarket proponents argue, we already allow the exchange of labor for wages, which actually consists of the sale of labor; if we tolerate prostitution, which consists of the hiring of the female body; if we permit paid experimentation with drugs using human beings—then why should we disapprove of or prohibit the buying and selling of organs, blood, and gametes?

The validity of these analogies is undeniable. In logical terms, however, the argument that "if certain forms of commerce of the human body are accepted, why not accept also the direct buying and selling of parts of the body?" may also be reversed. It could be argued that one of the reasons for considering the buying and selling of organs, tissues, gametes, and so on as immoral is that this could increase and consolidate other, more traditional forms of commerce in humans. However, the principal response to the analogy argument consists in exploring the substantial differences among the situations cited above.

Testing a medical treatment, not on volunteers or on patients who might benefit from it but on persons participating as the result of coercion (prisoners, the mentally handicapped, or persons in similar conditions), or else by recruiting subjects through offers of money, has long been considered ethically reprehensible. Even when permitted, a rule exists: experimentation must never cause irreversible damage. The removal of a kidney certainly does not satisfy this criterion. As for prostitution, it has always existed, practically everywhere in the world. In many cases, it has been legitimized by legislation, and even by religion, despite its representing a material and symbolic expression of male arrogance. In a large number of countries, however, the exploitation of the prostitute is considered a crime. The difference is that prostitution can take place in the absence of mediation, while the biotechnological market could not exist without the intervention of professional skills, specialized centers, and brokering techniques. Lastly, the analogy with the sale of labor is weaker than the others. What makes paid labor different from slave labor is that paid labor is temporary and discretionary. It is true that paid labor may be harmful and may jeopardize workers' lives. It is also true that the effect of the industrial revolution on workers in its early years has been described as "peaceful genocide," in view of the widespread suffering it caused. Later, however, conditions for workers in developed democratic countries began to improve, under the combined effects of inquiries, struggles, trade unions, legislation, and guaranteed rights. It is frightening to think that the biomarket could establish itself through a period of exploitation of the human body similar to that which accompanied the Industrial Revolution. It is also unimaginable that a balance of power similar to that existing to some extent between workers and capital—a balance that has led to substantial social progress in many parts of the world—could be attained in the biotechnological market, which necessarily involves isolated sellers. I have difficulty imagining that the sellers of their own body parts could be gathered together into organizations resembling trade unions and could succeed in gaining real bargaining power in negotiations with buyers backed by resources, associations, structures, and professional expertise. This wide gap between the power of buyer and seller is also seen in the fact that the subject receiving an organ transplant is scrupulously and regularly monitored and assisted after the operation, while nothing of the kind is offered to the so-called "paid donor."

After examining the analogies proposed, I was struck that no one has so far invoked *slavery* as a term of comparison for the biotechnological market. This ethically most significant and longest lasting experiment in the marketing of humans in history has been neglected, repressed. The reason for this silence may be that, today, slavery has become synonymous with barbarity. Therefore a comparison between slavery as unregulated commerce in human beings (including their descendants) and the biotechnological market of "separate parts" of the body would certainly create a deep spontaneous repulsion for biomarketing.

Slavery, however, also had its supporters, who justified it on practical and ethical grounds, so I deemed it of interest to examine the moral arguments put forward in defense of slavery in past centuries. I attempted to establish whether a comparison on the basis of analogies and differences could be made with the present arguments for and against the biotechnological market of human beings. There is no need to include here the documentation of the massacres and human rights violations accompanying slavery in both the ancient and the modern world, documentation especially complete for the seventeenth and eighteenth centuries, when slavery became an essential component in the colonization of the Americas and other continents and in the commercial and industrial progress of Europe. The facts have now been widely proved.

On an ethical plane, the use of the body as a commodity was based on the assumption that the human being can be evaluated as an object, like a capital asset. In the classical world the slave was considered an *instrumentum vocale;* that is how the ancients distinguished a slave from a tool, *instrumentum mutum,* and from an animal, *instrumentum semivocale.* The Old Testament contains no explicit declaration against slavery, and in ancient Greece the enslavement of foreigners was justified by their different natures. In the philosophical field, as David Brion Davis has amply demonstrated, "the legal and moral value of slavery represented an embarrassing problem for European thinkers from Aristotle to Locke." The problem became particularly acute in the eighteenth century, when "western thinking turned to history to seek moral guidance and a way of understanding," and the controversies over slavery in the Americas and over the organized trafficking of the European nations "occupied an important place in the classics of history and law, in economic policy and moral philosophy" (10, pp. 39–40).

The principle according to which all human beings have equal rights and thus the human body is *res non commerciabilis* was the firmest and most coherent moral basis of the abolitionist movements. The first restrictions to be placed on slave traffic were introduced in the eighteenth century. Towards the end of that century, the states of Pennsylvania and Massachusetts voted in favor of the gradual abolition of slavery; several years later, during the French Revolution, the Convention, keeping faith with the principles of justice and equality, approved by acclamation a similar decision (a decision later abrogated by Napoleon). International rules were introduced in the nineteenth century through several different agreements between countries; in the end, the Geneva Convention (September 26, 1926) decreed that all nations must "pursue the suppression of slavery in all its forms, as soon as possible."

JUSTIFICATIONS FOR SLAVERY

I have merely outlined the ideas that accompanied both slavery and the abolitionist movements and convinced the world that slavery was inhuman: Brion Davis and many others have provided a much wider range of ideas and documentation on both phases of this history. I endeavor here to discuss, for the purpose of making a comparison with the present-day biomarket, three arguments used in the past to justify slavery: its necessity for the common good, the benefits that slaves themselves derived from it, and the conditions deriving from slaves' perceived inferiority.

For the Common Good

One of the most frequently used arguments pointed out the advantages for the economy. Slavery, the argument ran, was essential, indispensable, and irreplaceable for the "common good." In 1688, for example, the French governor of Canada, Denonville, wrote to Louis XIV to request authorization to import black slaves directly from Africa, an enterprise he deemed indispensable to make up for the lack of labor power in Canada, and necessary for the prosperity of France. The attorney general, Ruette d'Auteil, persuaded the king, claiming that Africans, accustomed as they were to the deserts of Africa, would easily adapt to the "cold desert" (10, p. 159) of Canada. In 1709, a pamphlet published in London with the telling title *The Slave Trade, the Great Pillar and Support of the British Plantations in Africa,* put forward the claim that production in the colonies using slaves was an indispensable element of the trade system on which the British Empire was based. Fifty years later, another pamphlet stated that slave traffic had only one justification—economic necessity—and that "The impossibility of doing without slaves in the West Indies will always prevent this traffic being dropped" (quoted in 11).

Similar arguments are used on behalf of the biotechnology market. Scientific progress would be slowed without paid drug experimentation, disease research hindered without the authorization to patent human DNA, and the possibility of performing transplants hindered without the right to purchase organs taken from corpses and kidneys sold by living donors. The market, according to this argument, is the only way to resolve the gap between demand and supply. The expression "buy or die" implies that there is no alternative: in order to survive, one must buy and sell. Those who oppose the marketing of human organs commit an infringement of personal freedom and deny to patients on transplant waiting lists the chance to live. (In fact, however, in some countries, such as Spain, encouraging donations and organizing services appropriately has offset the imbalance between supply of and demand for organs.)

Two questions come to mind regarding these moral and practical problems of the past and present. First, to what extent has the "human market" been a cause not of growth but of stagnation and regression—that is, an obstacle to technological, scientific, and social development? As far as the past is concerned, it is not difficult to show that slavery has been a hindrance to progress. For example, some of the principles of physics on which modern technology is based were already known in ancient times, such as the invention by Hero of Alexandria of an apparatus that used a steam jet to move a wheel; but practical applications of these principles were not implemented for nearly 2,000 years, mainly because producing energy mechanically would be redundant in societies based on slavery. In the eighteenth and nineteenth centuries, figures such as David Hume, Adam Smith, and Benjamin Franklin—who, according to Burton M. Leiser, "did not see slavery as a fundamentally immoral institution, even when they opposed it"—criticized slavery mainly because they "simply believed that slavery was an inherently inefficient, expensive way to produce goods and services. In their view, slave societies inhibited population growth and therefore industrial progress and the scientific advances that industry brings in its wake. Because industry is essential to the production of wealth, societies that permit slavery were in their opinion more likely to be slower in accumulating wealth than those that relied on a free labor force" (12, p. 127). *A posteriori,* one might point out that the affirmation of human rights, of which the abolition of slavery was an essential part, coincided in the West with the maximum development of wealth, science, prosperity, and social justice.

Coming back to the present day, I am convinced that allowing human blood and organs to be bought and sold is not conducive to but rather an obstacle to donation. Very few persons are actually willing to donate when, along with the concept of solidarity towards all human beings, there is a free market in which those to be treated and those not, those who can live and those who must die, are selected according to their wealth. This market would also discourage the search for alternative solutions: increased donations; prevention of diseases that create the need for transplants; improved efficiency in the removal, storage, transport, and implantation of organs; and scientific research aimed at finding other solutions such as artificial blood and organs and xenotransplantation.

The second question is: can it be right, in response to impulses triggered by the needs of the moment, to waive the historical and ethical values that represent the fundamental components of our civilization? Slavery developed in a primitive context, but the rise of democratic civilization began precisely with *habeas corpus*. The right to autonomy of the body must be asserted not only against the abuse of political power but also against the totalizing power of the market. Bringing the fundamental freedoms into conflict through a distorted conception of "common good" is unacceptable; if this were to be allowed, both freedom and the common good would be sacrificed.

For the Victims' Good

The second argument advanced in favor of slavery, which attempted to reconcile interest in retaining slavery with compassion for its victims, was grounded in claims of the benefits for the slaves themselves. In his analysis of the "comparative defense of slavery" by those in the United States who were opposed to its abolition, Peter Kolchin asserts that the idea was current that, "far from being oppressed under slavery, Southern slaves receive unparalleled care and protection and were in fact better off than most supposedly free workers in Britain and the Northern United States" (13). Today, along the same lines, a transplant surgeon has claimed: "A poor starving Indian who sells a kidney to a rich Arab sheikh who is dying of uremia makes two persons happy."

"For love of the slaves" justifications were alternately spiritual and material. On the spiritual side, for example, we find the decree issued in 1363 by the priors of Florence, after plague and famine had decimated the population of the city. The decree authorized the importation of male and female slaves under one condition: they must not be Christians. The main argument was that this would make it possible to wrest infidels and idolaters from their native environments and bring them to Christian lands, thus saving their souls (14). On the material side, a more reasoned and complex explanation was set out in 1907 in the monumental book *Folkways,* in which Graham Sumner commented on the customs, way of life, and morals of different societies (15).With reference to slaves, he suggested that they were often happy in their condition. His claim was based on the fact that, in human history, slavery "began where the economic system was such that there was a gain in making a slave from a war captive instead of killing him." But in addition to the advantage of not being killed (and, I could add, eaten), slavery "proved to be a great schoolmaster in teaching men steady work." This was essential, as "no man would do any hard, persistent work if he could help it." The defeated, turned into slaves, were obliged to work hard and learned to accept slavery. They "helped the whole society up to a higher status, in which they also share. . . . They were proud of this slavery, proud of belonging to the 'cultivated' and of being 'wild' men no longer. In that view slavery is a part of the discipline by which the human race has learned how to carry on the industrial organization" (15).

In actual fact, gratitude for such benefits cannot have been so generalized or pride at being civilized so widespread, given that slave revolts, only sporadic at the beginning, from the eighteenth century arose regularly in many countries (especially in the Caribbean) and counted among the factors leading to slaves' liberation. Nevertheless, as late as 1996, Charles Davidson, a Republican senator from Alabama, in a speech delivered before the state parliament, claimed that slaves used to be better off, while now "the number of rapes, holdups and murders is a hundred times greater among the blacks living in ghettos than when they were slaves" (quoted in 16). He included in his speech a quotation from the Bible (Leviticus 25:39–46), according to which it was prohibited to make slaves of the "children of Israel" but permitted to "enslave the men and women of the surrounding nations."

To come back to the biotechnology market, contracts with "surrogate mothers" are allowed and, indeed, advertised in the United States—allowed both because they are legal and because they are deemed by some to be advantageous both for the adoptive parents and for the woman who agrees to carry through a pregnancy and then hand over the child she bears. Laws in many European nations prohibit such contracts or declare them to be null and void. The European Parliament has even prohibited the paid donation of blood (I note, however, that blood and plasma continue to be imported from third world countries; that is, from "surrounding nations," as allowed by the book of Leviticus).

The implications of this provision could be interpreted to mean that if we were to accept and update Sumner's arguments concerning the benefits of slavery, they could be paradoxically extended from the categories of blood, gametes, and organs to include the whole human body. Let us take an example. In the developed countries, there are more families wanting to adopt a child than children available for legal adoption. To allow children to be bought could bring solace to the impecunious parents who sell them and happiness to those who adopt them and—why not?—to many of the adopted children. It is highly probable, in fact, that children from the ex-colonies of Mozambique or Somalia, sold in Portugal or in Italy, would have a longer and better life than their peers remaining in the country of origin. Another example can be given. The developed countries have more insalubrious and unpleasant jobs than local workers willing to do them. To enlist slaves for the performance of these tasks would make the slave traders happy (as they were in the nineteenth century), the buyers happy, and also some of the sold workers happy, provided the contracts contained clauses guaranteeing some advantage over and above the few benefits they currently enjoy as "free immigrant workers." Many of the workers would in any case have a better life than in their own countries. This could also represent an advantage for the community and its social cohesion: immigrants to Europe from other continents, and Mexican immigrants to the United States, would most likely be much better accepted if they were to welcome voluntarily such a clearly defined status. Probably a few voices would be raised, in the spirit of John Stuart Mill: the principle of freedom cannot admit the freedom not to be free (17). But one could reply using Sumner's words: "A humanitarian doctrine which orders that a slave be turned out of doors, in spite of his own will, is certainly absurd" (15, pp. 305–306).

When the abolitionist movement developed, there was a parallel increase in the number of political and cultural initiatives and government decisions based on the idea that the "victims' good" could be pursued more effectively and less traumatically by means of "permit and protect" policies, aimed at regulating and humanizing slavery by guaranteeing a more humane treatment of slaves (18). During the second half of the eighteenth century, for example, the state of South Carolina diluted the legislative provisions that had allowed masters to kill or mutilate their slaves with impunity (10, p. 87). In the same period, the British government ordered that a physician should travel on board each slave ship together with its human cargo, and that the captain of the vessel should receive a prize for each slave delivered alive to his or her destination (19). And in the following century, the Portuguese government decreed the children of slave parents to be free (provided they served their masters until the age of 20).

Similar measures are proposed today to regulate and humanize the biotechnology market by means of incentives and inducements offered to those who sell parts of their body. For example, living persons who agree to make an organ donation are promised priority on waiting lists to receive transplants (at the same time, there is a proposal to exclude from such a list all those who declare themselves non-donors). Or parents of a deceased person are to be given prizes in the form of money, or insurance or reductions in public tariffs, or at least a free funeral for their dear ones, in exchange for authorization to use the deceased's organs. Numerous highly imaginative proposals have been advanced in this direction, often lacking not only in moral but in common sense, such as that of setting a fair price and, in Great Britain, of giving the National Health Service the monopoly of buying and selling organs (20).

Thus, permit and protect policies, although based on humanitarian intentions at the outset, actually lead to the transformation of the human body into a commodity or a reserve of spare parts. Between the cases of slavery and the biomarket, however, there is a very substantial difference. Slavery, at the time when its humanization was under discussion, was accepted practically everywhere. Its regulation, and the reduction or elimination of some of its crueler and more inhumane aspects, represented the first step towards its abolition. The biotechnology market, on the other hand, is, fortunately, comparatively restricted. Its legalization, whatever form it takes, can encourage its expansion.

The Inferiority of Slaves

To my mind, if we reject the arguments of the common good and of the benefits to the victims, the only way the use of humans as a commodity can be justified is by viewing a segment of humanity as subhuman or nonhuman and their bodies as at the disposal of others. This view is at the very heart of slavery, and those who champion it have looked to religious, cultural, and anthropological reasoning in its defense.

Noah's Biblical curse of Canaan as "slave of his brothers' slaves" (Genesis 9:25) was widely used in the eighteenth century to justify the conditions of Africans enslaved on the American continent. The same idea—that is, that to be a slave was the consequence of a sin—had been expressed by Isidore of Seville in the sixth century: "Slavery is a punishment meted out to humanity for the original sin" (21). For the abbot Smaragdus of Saint Michel, in the ninth century, slaves were the result not of nature but of a fault committed. And so on, down to very recent times. According to Burton M. Leiser, "the Church did not reject the support of slavery until the year 1965, with the resolutions of the Vatican II Council" (12, p. 127); however, this is probably too harsh a judgment, because it does not take into account Christ's message being intrinsically hostile to slavery, or the positive movements stemming from this inspiration. As Leiser himself notes, Aristotle claimed "that some persons are naturally inclined to be free while others are more inclined by nature to be slaves" (*Politics,* 1327B) and that there-fore "it is an advantage for them also to be slaves" (12, pp. 126–127). Lastly, Leiser cites the definition of the nature of Africans according to the 1797 edition of the *Encyclopaedia Britannica,* which lists their characteristics as "idleness, treachery, revenge, cruelty, impudence, stealing, lying, profanity, debauchery, nastiness and intemperance . . . they are strangers to every sentiment of com-passion, and are an awful example of the corruption of man when left to himself" (12, p. 127).

The anthropological argument was widely debated in Europe and America in the nineteenth century, before and after the American civil war, in, for example, the books *Indigenous Races of the Earth* and *Instincts of Races* (22, 23). The idea that people of African origin were biologically inferior implied a responsibility on the part of whites to look after them, to make them industrious and happy, so that as slaves they could have a better life and become more intelligent than those who remained in their original lands. These ideas circulated in Europe, in particular in the United Kingdom and France, giving rise to an extensive debate among anthropologists. This topic is analyzed, for example, in Jacque Roger's essay in *Histoire de l'anthropologie* (24).

Implicit in the theory of natural inferiority was the unacceptability and thus the need for punishment of sexual relations between white women and black men (though not between white men and black women, of course). To return to the present day, it is clear that the criterion of natural inferiority cannot be applied to organ transplants and blood transfusions—not, at least, since the heart of a black man was transplanted into a white by Christian Barnard in South Africa at the time of apartheid. Since then, the donation of blood and organs has revealed the total biological compatibility among the various human strains. However, the theory of inferiority has survived these scientific proofs, as well as many others of a cultural nature, and has had a considerable influence on the psychological characteristics, moral behavior, and developmental potential of "those that are different from us."

In any case, when the exchange of body parts is not regulated by availability of donations but by the market, another type of inferiority becomes dominant. I refer to the comparative wealth and power of buyers and sellers, which is no less significant and persistent than status determined by tradition, religion, and law. The truth of the matter is that, as far as human organs are concerned, the traffic always takes place between the South and the North of the world, or between the poor who sell and the rich who buy. We can therefore envisage a future scenario by following the implications of present arrangements, both for potential adoptees and for immigrant laborers, to their logical conclusions: in the twenty-first century, the North could attempt to treat its more seriously ill by importing and using organs removed from members of the poorer classes, in particular from the underdeveloped countries. Supplies would be more than sufficient, as bodies are the only goods that these countries produce in abundance. It would be tragically ironic, having first contributed through development of biomedical science to improvements in the lives of residents of remote lands, to bring them to the biomarket in order to harvest their vital organs.

PRESENT-DAY FORMS OF SLAVERY

My main ethical concern, however, is not this gloomy prospect, which I have presented in a paradoxical manner and which is in any case certainly avoidable. My concern stems from the simultaneous presence of two parallel phenomena: the persistence or growth of the human market in the form of slavery, and the extension of the biomarket towards new "objects" that, immediately after (or even before) technical and scientific progress makes them available, are rapidly included in the catalogue of marketable goods. Slavery and biomarket coexist and are interwoven in our times, times in which the contrast between the expansion of proclaimed rights and the drama of violated rights is there for all to see.

This clash of the theoretical and the actual was brutally impressed upon me in 1996, on an air trip to the city of Fortaleza, in northeast Brazil, to deliver an address at the sixteenth National Conference of the Association of Lawyers. I was delighted at the opportunity, as I recalled memorable legal battles for human rights guided by the Association during the years of the military dictatorship. Nevertheless, I was surprised at the invitation, never having been a lawyer, or a defendant, or even a witness in legal proceedings. However, the request did not lie entirely outside my area of competence: I was asked to talk about the right to health, because the theme of the conference was "the new rights": these included the environment, information, personal security, consumer protection, and health. I got an inkling of abuses of rights to come while observing the passengers in the aircraft taking us from Europe to Brazil and overhearing fragments of their conversations: they were all middle-aged men, traveling alone. I guessed that they would be finding company at Fortaleza and surroundings. After I landed, my Brazilian friends, to my great shame, explained to me that my interpretation was correct and that this, their destination, was noted for its profusion of locations where the recruitment of minors as prostitutes took place.

This is one of the forms of modern slavery. Commenting on a UNICEF report on the sexual exploitation of 8- to 16-year-old children that occurs in various parts of the world, Anna Oliverio Ferraris wrote, "Not only are many of them doomed to early death from AIDS, but they also suffer very violent traumas that mark them for the rest of their lives. Deprived of freedom and their childhood, they are placed at the mercy of pedophile tourists from various countries, including Italy: these tourists exploit their wretched economic and moral conditions to do what they would not be allowed to do at home, using third-world children as 'disposable objects,' as commodities that may be legitimately consumed" (25).

Commenting on the laws aimed at putting an end to the sexual exploitation of children, Bharati Sadasivam wrote that they "are characterized by timid half measures and ambiguity and reflect the capitulation of many governments before the blandishments of the tourist industry, before the powerful interests of organized crime and the commodification of women in the popular mass media" (26).

Minors' rights have also been constantly discussed for at least ten years with reference to two other conditions. One is war: "the compulsory recruitment of children for military service and its serious consequences has been denounced in many parts of the world. Many are killed or taken prisoner, others are interrogated, tortured, beaten, or kept as prisoners of war" (27). Recruitment of children for war takes place, above all, in poor countries, as a part of conflicts unleashed by local powers and interests and fought using weapons purchased from the rich countries. The other condition is labor: a document written for the U.N. human rights campaign explains that child labor is used because it is "cheap" and because children "are naturally more docile and easier to discipline than adults, and are afraid to complain." For these reasons, work is often given to children while their parents remain jobless. Exploitation of child labor is often linked to multinational corporations that transfer their labor-intensive activities abroad, especially those activities that require simple repetitive work rather than knowledge, and that locate part of their production in poorer, more permissive countries.

In recent years the conscience of people living in the rich countries, who find themselves consuming high-quality products processed by children working in inhuman conditions, has been somewhat troubled by this contradiction. Opinion movements and associations have emerged, such as the Fair Trade Organization and TransFair, an international body that certifies the fair origin, untainted by child labor, of products coming from the South and sold on the market in the North. Trade unions, particularly those in the United States, have also addressed this problem and made it a central point in their political opposition at the Seattle meeting of the World Trade Organization. Their opposition has received both approval and criticism; the former owing to the appeal to worldwide worker solidarity, the latter owing to the suspicion that they were trying to protect themselves from competition and prevent the development, in whatever form, of the poor countries. This situation, with its manifold complex and tormented ethical facets, has finally been brought to the world's attention.

Thus far in my treatment of present-day slavery I have dwelt on children, but there are many other conditions that cry out for discussion. The World Labor Report published in 1993, for example, dedicated its first chapter to an alarmed description and cataloguing of the various forms of forced labor in existence today: traditional slavery (Mauritania and Sudan); bonded labor, in which a worker is bound to a company for life by inextinguishable debts (Pakistan, India, Peru); the forced labor of persons who are uprooted, transferred, and forced to work under the threat of arms (Brazil, Dominican Republic); compulsory chores on behalf of a community; the delivery of convicts as labor to private companies; and servile labor of minors (28). For the specifically female forms of forced labor, I could also cite as evidence the documentation of the Fourth U.N. World Conference on Women (Peking, 1995) and the subsequent updates on this problem (e.g., 29). The picture is an alarming one and justifies the somber tone of the final statement in the report: "At the end of the twentieth century many believe that slavery has been eradicated. Unfortunately it has not."

These reports also illustrate the progress made in many countries, as well as in the drafting of international charters and national legislation. However, there is an increasingly evident contradiction between recognized rights and the institutions set up to implement them in everyday practice. The plethora of proclamations and the huge number of international organizations (U.N. and ILO for labor; WHO for health; UNESCO for education and culture; FAO for food; UNICEF for children; U.N. Commission for Women, etc.) often appear as a superstructure covering up rather than revealing, preventing, punishing, and remedying these cases of extreme exploitation.

THE NEW "OBJECTS" OF THE BIOMARKET

The same contradiction is beginning to emerge in the biotechnology market. I do not want to undervalue, in an atmosphere in which the market tends to overwhelm all other values, the WHO declaration against the sale of organs and parts of the human body or the UNESCO declaration on the human genome, approved "unanimously and by acclamation" on November 11, 1997. The latter, after stating that the genome is symbolically the property of humanity and that the dignity of individuals "requires that individuals not be reduced to their genetic characteristics and [should receive] respect for the unique nature of each one as well as their diversity," proclaims (Article 4) that "the human genome in its natural state cannot be a source of profit." By the time this declaration was approved, however, patents had already been filed for more than 2000 genes (U.S. National Institutes of Health); requests for patents, filed by numerous applicants, have since increased exponentially.

In addition, Article 21 of the Bioethical Convention approved by the Council of Europe (30) states, "The human body and its parts must not as such represent a source of profit." Crystal clear, like the UNESCO formulation. Unfortunately, the European Parliament then approved Directive no. 44/98/EC (31) (challenged by Holland and Italy in the International Court), which is in complete contradiction with this policy. Article 5, after solemnly stating that the mere discovery of a sequence or a partial sequence of a gene "cannot constitute a patentable invention," allows for an exception of unlimited scope when the discovery is made "by means of a technical procedure."

How is it possible, I wonder, to isolate a gene sequence without using a technical procedure? During my zigzagging scientific activities, I was for many years a parasitologist, working on living material much larger than genes, from protozoa upwards. In order to examine malaria plasmodia, I had to smear a drop of infected blood on a slide, stain it, and then observe the plasmodia under the microscope. To see whether there were any worm eggs in human feces, I had to centrifuge a specimen, and I swear it was not a pleasant "technical procedure." Even in identifying fleas, to discover, for example, whether they have a hair in front of or below the eye (a fact of no aesthetic interest, but used to distinguish a species capable of transmitting the plague from another, harmless species), I had to give them successive treatments with potassium hydrate, phenol, cedar oil, xylol, and Canadian balsam before pressing them delicately between two slides; otherwise, I would not have been able to see much even under the microscope (summarized from the "Rosicky method," 32; see also 33). I have asked many geneticists whether technical procedures are necessary to identify gene sequences, and they have all answered yes—but, of course, much more sophisticated procedures.

In an attempt to reconcile ethical principles with industrial and commercial interests, the European Union resorts to hypocrisy and the United States to legal subtleties. In 1984, as soon as transplants were seen to be successful and the commercial use of organs could be envisaged, Congress passed the National Organ Transplant Act, which punishes the sale of organs with fines and prison sentences. However, the law does not cover blood, because it is not considered an organ; spermatozoa and ova are not included, because they are considered cells, and to hire a uterus because it is temporary in nature. Trade in these items is flourishing, especially over the Internet. At the Web site www.ronsangels.com, for example, one can purchase the ova of top models selected on the basis of their photographs; at www.geniusspermbank.com, the sperm of men with a very high IQ (the sperm bank of Nobel prize winners, set up in 1983, has unfortunately closed down). And the Creating Families site, www.creat-fam.com/home.htm, contains a huge stable of surrogate mothers (34). The latter "business" is probably the one with the greatest similarity to slavery, for two reasons. First, newborns are purchased by client couples through a delivery contract negotiated with the pregnant woman, a contract that U.S. jurisprudence deems more binding than the ties of maternity (thus giving the monetary relationship priority over the natural relationship). In Italy and elsewhere, however, the Civil Code states that the newborn is the child of the mother who gave birth to it. Second, the pregnant woman is, for nine months, no longer free: she is in fact obliged by contract to observe constraining rules of behavior, treatment, and tests, to ensure that the "product" is delivered in the best possible condition at birth.

Another feature of U.S. bioethical regulations is that they accept and legitimize the existence of a dual ethics. Very few laws are, like the Transplant Act, valid *erga omnes*. The majority of such laws are not valid for all, but only for institutions receiving federal funding. Thus, for example, the presidential decrees banning the production of embryos for experimental purposes or for sale or for the cloning of human beings are in no way binding on institutions funded by private enterprise or by the various states, all of which can operate without any limitations. Given this current legal arrangement, I have tried to imagine a possible chain of events. A biotechnology company produces human embryos by *in vitro* fertilization; it multiplies them by exploiting the property of early embryonic cells, each cell producing a new embryo; it patents them and sells them on the domestic and international markets, ready for different uses: for experimentation, for drug production, or (as sufficiently sophisticated incubators still do not exist) to be raised as clones by surrogate mothers—all in complete compliance with legal strictures. I presented this hypothesis as a question (at the Journées d'éthique, organized by the French Bioethics Committee, Paris, December 15, 1999) to Professor A. Capron, member of the National Advisory Bioethics Committee appointed by President Clinton—is such a chain of events possible? The answer was yes. The pathway to the patenting of embryos has also been opened by the European Patent Office, which has authorized the patenting of "embryos of mammals, including the human species." Each country, of course, has the right to pass its own laws. On a few, very few, issues, however, the idea is emerging of proceeding towards laws with universal application—as was the case in the past for slavery.

CAN THE TREND BE REVERSED?

We should be aware that, at the beginning of the new century, a high degree of alarm exists in many parts of the world, including the developed countries, at the persistence of archaic forms and growth of new forms of slavery. I am not sure whether these new forms of slavery are emerging at a faster rate than was the case in the past or are simply rendered more visible by the media and other forms of communication. What is certain is that being aware of them today implies shouldering political and moral responsibilities at the world level. We should also consider that, for the first time in history, current generations are faced with the possibility of being able to use their own body parts, which may represent either an extremely noble expression of the synergy between science and solidarity or else a biotechnical form of human exploitation.

It is no coincidence that the discussion on the patentability of genes is a problem for nations; that human cloning gives rise to wide-ranging scientific, philosophical, and religious controversies; and that in some quarters the question has been asked, "what is wrong with slavery?" (35). At the same time, we seek a "counterposition between economic and technical-scientific competition and ethical needs" (36) and ask whether (and which) fundamental rules may be invoked to reverse the trend towards the commodification of human beings.

I do not claim to be able to answer these questions. Perhaps a good approach would be to step back, to return to a discussion in Sumner's *Folkways,* written in the early twentieth century (15). Sumner's initial statement, which I consider both correct and significant because it underlines the important role that culture and ethics can play, is a comment on the abolition of slavery: "It is the only case in the history of mores where the so-called moral motive has been made controlling." But his following argument attempts to contradict the rightness of this historical achievement:

> In South Africa and in our own southern states the question of sanitary and police control is arising to present a new difficulty. . . . Are free men free to endanger peace, order, and health? Is a low and abandoned civilization free to imperil a high civilization, and entitled to freedom to do so? The humanitarians of the nineteenth century did not settle anything. The contact of two races and two civilizations cannot be settled by any dogma. Evidence is presented every day that problems are not settled and cannot be settled by any dogma. Is it not a sentiment made ridiculous when it is offered as a rule of action to a man who does not understand and does not respond to it?

His final statement is that "slavery is an interest that overwhelms all restrictions and all rules" (15, p. 306).

Similar arguments are put forward for today's biomarket: the law of competition will inexorably overwhelm all rules; appeals to "generic and sentimental dogmas" are pointless; any limit to experiments on humans "jeopardizes civilization" and will certainly obstruct advances beneficial to health. I would say, however, that at the practical level the events of the twentieth century, even with all their torments and tragedies, disproved rather than confirmed the gloomy forecasts made by Sumner at its beginning.

Examining the ethical implications of this question, R. M. Hare recently asked, "What is wrong with slavery?" (35). In answer he presented a number of scenarios, including one in which large populations of slaves maintain a high standard of living for a minority (an arrangement most would consider, as Hare says, totally unjustifiable), and another in which a small number of slaves are considered necessary for the good of the majority (a hypothesis, Hare suggests, that could enlist some justification). He goes on to examine arguments based both on principles (e.g., each person has equal value) and on consequences, which show "through the study of history and other factual observations, that slavery does have the effects (namely the production of misery) which make it wrong." He concludes, "I would always vote for the abolition of slavery, even though I would admit that cases could be *imagined* in which slavery would do more good than harm, and even though I am an utilitarian" (35, pp. 179, 180).

In the biomarket there is also another consequential issue, which derives from a fundamental difference from slave traffic. Slavery demanded of its promoters and organizers only an enterprising spirit undaunted by violence; the biomarket demands the active participation of qualified professionals with expertise in many scientific fields, professionals who may be diverted from other work with unambiguously humanitarian aims. Dorothy Nelkin and Lori Andrews wrote that the transformation of the human body into a commodity "violates body integrity, exploits powerless people, intrudes on community values, distorts research agendas, and weakens public trust in scientists and clinicians" (37).

These ethical questions would become even more serious if a chapter of history introducing human cloning were to open—that is, the production of predetermined human beings. If the cloning of humans were allowed, it would be difficult to avoid new forms of subordination for human beings designed to possess particular characteristics or, perhaps, modified to perform specific functions. The birth of cloned humans resistant to radiation or to chemical agents has already been envisaged; from there, it is a short step to their duplication for use in factories or other contaminated areas that would be highly hazardous for ordinary human beings. The old Aristotelian idea that slavery is a natural consequence of natural differences (after ideas of slavery based purely on race have become obsolete) would receive a new lease of life; and if natural differences were somehow found insufficient, no matter: biotechnology could create new ones.

REFERENCES

1. Crawford, C. Between Contract and Charity: Patients' Rights and Clinical Trials in Eighteenth Century England. Paper presented at the Conference on Coping with Sickness, Health, and Human Rights: An Historical Perspective, Castelvecchio Pascoli, March 1997.
2. Beauchamp, T. L., and Faden, R. R. History of informed consent. In *Encyclopedia of Bioethics,* edited by W. T. Reich, vol. 3, pp. 1233–11234. Simon & Schuster, New York, 1995.
3. Plato. Le leggi. In *Opere,* vol. 2, p. 715. Laterza, Bari, 1967.
4. La legge e il corpo (special issue). *Democrazia e diritto* 36(1), January-March 1996.
5. Shorter, E. *Storia del corpo femminile.* Feltrinelli, Milan, 1984 (*A History of Women's Bodies,* Basic Books, New York, 1982).
6. *Proceedings of the European Parliament,* Session of September 13, 1993, p. 20.

7. Porter, D. Preparing for the twenty-first century (Part 4). In *Health, Civilization, and the State: A History of Public Health from Ancient to Modern Times,* pp. 279–319. Routledge, London, 1999.

8. Berlinguer, G., and Garrafa, V. *La merce finale: Saggio sulla compravendita di parti del corpo umano.* Baldini e Castoldi, Milan, 1996.

9. Berlinguer, G., and Garrafa, V. *L'uomo in vendita.* Baldini e Castoldi, Milan, 2000.

10. Brion Davis, D. *Il problema della schiavitù nella cultura occidentale.* SEI, Turin, 1971 (*The Problem of Slavery in Western Culture,* Cornell University Press, Ithaca, 1966).

11. Coupland, A. *The British Anti-Slavery Movement,* p. 37. Thornton Butterworth, London, 1933.

12. Leiser, B. M. Slavery. In *Encyclopedia of Applied Ethics,* edited by R. Chadwick, vol. 4. Academic Press, San Diego, 1998.

13. Kolchin, P. *American Slavery,* p. 194. Penguin, London, 1995.

14. Origo, I. Presentazione. In *Il problema della schiavitù nella cultura occidentale,* by D. Brion Davis, p. 11. SEI, Turin, 1971 (*The Problem of Slavery in Western Culture,* Cornell University Press, Ithaca, 1966).

15. Sumner, W. G. *Folkways: A Study of the Sociological Importance of Usages, Manners, Customs, Mores, and Morals.* Ginn and Company, Boston, 1907.

16. *L'Unità,* May 5, 1996.

17. Stuart Mill, J. *Saggio sulla libertà,* p. 118. EST, Milan, 1997 (*The Collected Works of John Stuart Mill,* Toronto-London, 1963–1991).

18. Smith, W. H. *A Political History of Slavery,* vol. 1, p. 287. New York, 1903.

19. Balladore Pallieri, G. Schiavitù. In *Enciclopedia Italiana,* vol. 31, p. 86. Istituto Giovanni Treccani, Rome, 1929.

20. Lockwood, M. La donazione non altruistica di organi in vita. In *Questioni di Bioetica,* edited by S. Rodotà, pp. 139–147. Laterza, Bari, 1993.

21. Bloch, M. Come finí la schiavitù antica. In *Lavoro e tecnica nel medioevo,* p. 216. Laterza, Bari, 1959.

22. Nott, J. C., and Gliddon, G. R. *Indigenous Races of the Earth.* Lippincott, Philadelphia, 1857.

23. Nott, J. C. *Instincts of Races.* L. Graham, New Orleans, 1866 (reprinted in *New Orleans Med. Surg. J.*).

24. Roger, J. Buffon, Jefferson et l'homme américain. In *Histoire de l'anthropologie: Hommes, idées moments,* edited by C. Blanckaert, A. Ducros, and J. J. Hublin, pp. 57–66. Bulletin et Mémoires de la Société d'anthropologie de Paris, Paris, 1989.

25. Oliverio Ferraris, A. Fermiamo il commercio dei piccoli schiavi. *Corriere Salute,* January 9, 1995, p. 1.

26. Sadasivam, B. Dopo Pechino. In *Social Watch,* pp. 75–80. Rosenberg & Sellier, Turin, 1999.

27. United Nations. *Derechos humanos. Formas contemporàneas de la esclavitud.* Folleto informativo no. 14. Geneva, 1991.

28. International Labor Office. *World Labor Report 1993,* pp. 1–2, 9–18. Geneva, 1993.

29. Stern, J. Le donne nel mondo del lavoro: che ne è dell'impegno assunto? In *Social Watch,* pp. 75–80. Rosenberg & Sellier, Turin, 1999.

30. Council of Europe. *Convention for the Protection of Human Rights and Dignity of Human Beings with Regards to the Applications of Biology and Medicine: Convention on Human Rights and Biomedicine.* Strasbourg, November 19, 1996.

31. European Union. *Sulla protezione giuridica delle invenzioni biotecnologiche.* EC Official Gazette no. 90. Brussels, November 16, 1998.
32. Berlinguer, G. *Aphaniptera d'Italia: Studio monografico,* p. 40. Il Pensiero Scientifico, Rome, 1964.
33. Berlinguer, G. *Le mie pulci,* 2nd ed. Edizioni Studio Tesi, Pordenone, 1995.
34. Gabaglio, L. Voglio un bimbo.com. *L'Espresso,* May 18, 2000, pp. 149–156.
35. Hare, R. M. What is wrong with slavery? In *Applied Ethics,* edited by Peter Singer, pp. 165–183. Oxford University Press, Oxford, 1986.
36. Hottois, G. Il corpo e il mercato. In *Frontiere della vita,* vol. 4, p. 789. Istituto della Enciclopedia italiana, Rome, 1999.
37. Nelkin, D., and Andrews, L. Homo Economicus: Commercialization of body tissues in the age of biotechnology. *Hastings Center Rep.,* September-October 1998, p. 31.

CHAPTER 5

Global Health

WHY GLOBAL?

There may be some confusion about the meaning of "global health." For some it may mean complete health, the absence of all disease, defect, or imperfection. This utopian interpretation received some credit in the definition coined by the World Health Organization, according to which health is "a state of complete physical, mental and social well-being," a definition that has contributed to extending (too much, on occasion) the often purely organicist horizons of biomedicine. In the corridors of the WHO in Geneva, however, you occasionally hear someone muttering, "If someone came here and claimed to be in a state of complete well-being, etc., etc., we would have him put away in a mental institution." In fact, health is not a state and is not perfection. It is a condition of changeable equilibrium, which we can now, unlike in the past, shift considerably in a positive direction. But I think it highly unlikely that human perfection can be attained through hygiene and medicine; sometimes such attempts lead people to commit excesses and nations to commit abuses.

By "global health" I instead refer to the health of all human subjects, and I find valid reasons for placing this concept at the center of bioethical reflection on the relationship between health and disease. The main reason is that health, simultaneously one of the most intimate processes at the individual level and a process most closely linked to community life, has a dual value on the moral plane: *intrinsic,* as the presence, limitation, or absence of vital capacity (ultimately, as the antithesis between life and death), and *instrumental,* as an essential condition for living a free life. Freedom is indeed substantially impaired when disease prevails, (*a*) because the individual is usually hindered in one or more of her faculties of decision-making or action; (*b*) because her destiny is entrusted to external powers, especially when, as a sick person, she is no longer considered a citizen with rights; and (*c*) because disease, when serious and persistent, often leads the individual (and the nation) into downward mobility, into the vicious circle of a regression that may become irreversible. This has happened many times in the past and is happening again. For many Chinese peasants, for example, since the cutbacks or abolition of public health, sickness has become the main cause of a plunge into poverty, as was the case in Europe's rural areas one or two centuries ago. Several

African countries, struggling with hardships that include AIDS, poverty, and being more or less ignored by the rest of the world, have fallen into a crisis that will be hard to reverse.

I use "global health" also because health is an indivisible good. Humankind, as I shall attempt to show, is linked in the field of health by a common destiny. It is paradoxical, given today's all-pervasive globalization—of finance, instantaneous information, population migration, transfer of goods, production, consumption, human labor, organized crime, power systems, and scientific knowledge and technology—that an essential good such as health should be neglected or debased. Precisely because globalization constitutes the present and future phase of development, and because it can satisfy many human needs, we must address health as a global aim, as a good towards which all sides should be working in an explicit and planned way. The global dimension of health and of its associated moral choices is not, however, completely new; in different forms, it has existed throughout the centuries of the "modern era."

Even more than in the last chapter, I take a diachronic approach here in considering events and trends as they have occurred on the world scene. I thus endeavor to describe various phases in the form of a prologue followed by four acts, each with its own characteristics and its own moral coordinates. In the final discussion I consider the crucial topic of equity in health, the present trends towards globalization, and the accompanying moral choices.

PROLOGUE: MICROBIAL UNIFICATION
OF THE WORLD

The globalization of disease—that is, the spread of the same disease patterns worldwide—began in 1492 with the discovery (or conquest) of America. This marked the transition of populations, and thus of their diseases, from separation to global communication (1, 2). Even earlier in history, epidemic diseases had spread from one part of the world to another, following the migration of populations and trade; for instance, the plague and cholera traveled several times from Asia to Europe. However, before 1492, widely different conditions—determined by environment, nutrition, social and cultural organization, and, above all, the presence or absence of germs, biological vectors, and infectious diseases (everywhere the main cause of death)—had led to widely different epidemiological patterns in the new and old worlds. For example, America had no smallpox, measles, yellow fever, or malignant malaria, and probably no diphtheria, chicken pox, typhoid fever, scarlet fever, or influenza; Eurasia and Africa, no syphilis—a long list and a short one. And for this reason, the impact of new diseases after 1492 was devastating, especially on the American continent, whose populations had no immune defenses against the old world diseases. This, obviously, was an unpredictable and uncontrollable phenomenon and thus lies outside all moral judgment. Humans had neither the knowledge nor the means to take effective action, and in no way can we attribute "epidemic virginity"—that is, the unfavorable balance between the aggressiveness of the germs and the absence of any natural antibodies against them—to neglect or misconduct. Antibodies have always been the result of a long period of selection, coexistence, struggle, and adaptation between microorganism and host; only much later could antibodies be created as a product of science.

Nevertheless, other aspects of what happened in the new world do require ethical consideration. These stem from the contemporaneity of and synergism between the spread of disease, uncontrollable at the time, and the loss of identity, security, and power among the peoples of the American continent, the result of deliberate extermination, deadly slave labor in mines, breakdown in the food balance, and a psychological and cultural collapse that helped weaken resistance to disease and even led to an outbreak of suicides. The first, comprehensive denunciation of the "very long history of slaughter and devastation that could and should be drawn up" was written by Bishop Bartolomeo de Las Casas in 1552 (3). The most detailed analyses are those carried out during the closing decades of the twentieth century, under the influence of a radical historiographic reappraisal of the "Columbian exchange" (4; see also 5, 6). Over the four intervening centuries, the prevailing judgment on these phenomena adhered to the tradition of "history written by the winners," in at least two aspects. The first, found in every textbook, is the almost exclusive emphasis on disease, with a tendency to push into the background (and this is not the only example!) other causes of the slaughter that were deliberate and due to human fault. The other is the underestimation of the population losses on the American continent. The decrease in population during the sixteenth century was first estimated at "only" 5 to 10 million. Later research showed that in 1492 the Americas had a population equivalent to that of Europe (50 to 80 million); by the end of the sixteenth century no more than 10 million inhabitants remained. Even if this cannot in the strictest sense be defined as genocide, since the extermination was the result of a combination of natural causes and human decisions, it was certainly the greatest demographic tragedy experienced by the human species.

If we analyze the anthropological and ethical aspects of this experience, we encounter two myths that, together with ignorance about the causes and paths of diseases, have for many centuries conspired to hinder any human action to prevent and remedy the spread of disease. The first myth was the divine origin of disease: an expression of divine anger towards some or preference for other human beings. "When the Christians were left exhausted by the war," narrates Francisco de Aguilar, a follower of Cortés, "God decided to visit smallpox upon the Indians and a great pestilence broke out in the city." And on May 22, 1634, John Winthrop, first governor of the Massachusetts Bay Colony, noted, "As for the natives, they have practically all died of smallpox; in this way the Lord decided to clarify our right to what we possess" (both quoted in 7). It must be added that the same divine intervention was recognized by the American Indians themselves to explain the immunity of the Spanish to the evil that was exterminating the natives, which also contributed to the psychological collapse and defeat of the native peoples. The whole of scientific medicine, from Hippocrates onward, was built upon refuting this myth through its refusal to acknowledge the direct and personal presence of the divine in nature; its denial of the belief that epilepsy, for example, was a sacred illness: "As for the sacred illness, this is the truth. In no way is it more divine that the other diseases or more sacred, but it has a natural structure and rational causes" (8, p. 271).

The other myth attributed the origin of disease to the "enemy" or to some different, hostile, and suspect alien. This legend arose on the other side of the Atlantic, when syphilis broke out in Europe. Originating in the new world, this disease first appeared in Europe in epidemic form in 1495, during the siege and conquest of Naples by the French troops of Charles VIII. It hit the two armies in equal measure, although the Italians immediately called it "mal franzes" (or in more learned terms, *morbus gallicus*) and the French, "mal napolitain." When it reached the East, the Japanese dubbed it "Portuguese disease," and so on, each country blaming other nationalities. Twelve different "denominations of origin" have been recorded for syphilis, all unverified but stigmatizing, by the same number of populations and countries. Of course, when it became apparent that the disease originated in the Americas, the opportunity was not missed to blame the Indians—as victims of the disease because they "had not known the word of Christ" and as spreaders of the disease because of their "particularly lecherous habits" (9) (in enjoyment of which Columbus's sailors were known to be particularly refractory!). However, both before and after syphilis, the tendency to blame "others" for epidemics has been a constant feature in the history of disease. The Jews were blamed for carrying the black plague to Europe; the Irish, cholera to New York; the Italians, poliomyelitis to Brooklyn. Lastly, we should not forget that the first name given to AIDS by the U.S. Centers for Disease Control (CDC) was gay-related immune deficiency, as the first epidemic foci had been reported among the gay population; the blame was later laid on the Haitians. Epidemiological investigation must never neglect places, foci, environments, and behaviors likely to contribute to the spread of disease, but it is precisely legends like those described here that stand in the way of research.

ACT I: HEALTH POLICY BECOMES INTERNATIONAL

After the microbial unification of the globe, nearly three centuries were to pass before humankind (populations, governments, culture, and science) realized the common risks and began to make cross-border efforts to tackle them. These were not obscure centuries, however. The early seventeenth century saw the rise of scientific knowledge and experimentation. In the eighteenth century it was acknowledged that "saving souls is no longer the exclusive duty of families and of the lay and religious authorities. Saving bodies is an equally important task" (10), and giant strides were made in acknowledging that "the supernatural competence of the judge of souls, theologian and confessor, spiritual father and exorcist" must be "replaced by the natural judgment of morbid influences of the soul on the body and by the physician's skill" (11, pp. 83–84). Only in the nineteenth century, however, did the three essential premises for any effective action against disease come together: knowledge of the causes, identification of preventive and therapeutic remedies, and the will to take international action. The first confirmation that effective action was possible occurred in the late eighteenth century: the worldwide distribution of smallpox vaccine. Vaccination against smallpox had long been practiced in Asia, using serum drawn from healed smallpox blisters. Europe learned of the practice via Turkey, where female healers succeeded in inducing a mild form of the disease in children, thus giving them permanent immunity. Slaves, who had learned of the technique in Africa, introduced the same empirical knowledge into the new world. However, vaccination became common in Europe, then the rest of the world, only when Jenner—who also drew upon popular female experience—reinvented and perfected it and when, after promoting experimentation on convicts and orphan children, the British royal family agreed to be inoculated and thus encouraged the practice.

Two reasons why vaccination took such a long time to catch on in Europe are worth examining more closely. One reason lies in the "epistemological blindness" and professional haughtiness of European physicians, who were convinced they had nothing to learn from persons whom their prejudices led them to consider intellectually inferior on three grounds: as women, as quack doctors, and as Turks. The second reason resides in the theological debate on the very principle of vaccination. On one side where those opposed to vaccination on the grounds that it conflicted with the designs of divine providence, the sole arbiter of life, illness, and death (to which a double "specific aggravating circumstance" was added: that vaccine was an invention of Turkish infidels, spread throughout Europe by the physicians of Protestant England). On the other side were those who justified vaccination, again in the name of the same divine providence. In Italy considerable publicity was given to the opinion of three well-known Tuscan theologians who claimed that, despite what the enemies of vaccination were saying, it was those who refused vaccination and thus jeopardized human lives who were defying God, because the Lord teaches us to serenely accept diseases from his hand, but does not prohibit our taking precautions against them (12, cited in 13). The battle was also fought using the weapon of biblical quotations: "Non tentabis Dominum Deum tuum" versus "Honora medicum propter necessitatem, etenim illum creavit Altissimus" ("You will not tempt God, your Lord" versus "Honor the physician out of necessity, since he was created by the Lord on High"). Fortunately, medicine prevailed in the end.

Later, at the crossroad between the view of disease and suffering as a gift from God and the will to use medical science to assist the afflicted, after some soul-searching, the Catholic Church often opted for the more humanitarian path, following its tradition of charity and contributing to the spread of solidarity. The period of greatest progress in the struggle against epidemic diseases spanned the decades between the nineteenth and twentieth centuries, with discovery of the role of microbes in widespread and lethal infections such as tuberculosis, the plague, and cholera and of their paths of transmission via arthropod vectors or contaminated food and water. Sera and vaccines were introduced. Many infected cities were rehabilitated. Laws were passed to reduce the working day from 12 or 14 hours to 8 hours, to provide guarantees for pregnant women, and to limit children's work. The idea arose that, although the free market was a decisive factor in the progress of the economy, certain subjectss must be kept out of the market: human beings, in the first instance, because otherwise everyone's security and dignity would be jeopardized. Thus nations formulated national labor laws and universal rules against slavery. Social insurance and other forms of collective health protection became widespread, promoted or guaranteed by the actions of nation states. Lastly, nations entered into agreements on controlling the transmission of diseases from one part of the world to another.

The first steps in this direction were taken at the International Health Conference of 1851, attended by 11 European countries and Turkey. At this time, the geography of the more serious epidemics (cholera, the plague, and yellow fever) was known, but not their causes and the ways in which they were transmitted. The will to act thus preceded scientific certainty. Only 40 years and many conferences later (the seventh, in Venice in 1892) was a limited agreement reached on quarantine for ships arriving in Europe from the East. One reason for this delay was the opposition, especially by the British, to any rules that would hinder trade. This issue—the conflict between the free market and health measures, between priority accorded to profit and that accorded to health—had already arisen in Renaissance Tuscany (14) and continued to appear in new forms, with one side or the other prevailing or with more or less reasonable compromises imposed. The other reason for the delay in adopting international anti-epidemic measures was the scientific conflict between "miasma theory" and "contagion theory"—the two hypotheses on the origin and spread of epidemics that remained rivals until the end of the nineteenth century. By the time the Office International d'Hygiène Publique was set up in Paris (in 1907, with the agreement of 23 European countries), the discovery of microbes as infecting agents had essentially resolved this conflict. The contagion theory (first suggested by Girolamo Fracastoro in 1546, in his book *De contagione et contagiosis morbis* and in his hypothesis on germs, known as *seminaria prima*) finally triumphed, thanks to Pasteur, Koch, and other scientists. The scientific debate almost immediately became bound up with decision-making on health policy, and the latter with various moral questions. One of the most controversial issues was the relative influence of microbes and of the environment, nature, and culture in the origin and spread of disease (replacing the word "microbe" with "gene" would bring us to the present day). For instance, in Italy there was bitter controversy between the two great malariologists, Giovanni Battista Grassi and Angelo Celli. Grassi tended to reduce the pathogenic cycle to the equation: sick man plus *anopheles* equals malaria. Celli added to this equation other factors that were decisive in malarial epidemiology, such as living and working conditions, water supplies, food, and education; and he claimed that to combat the disease, the combined efforts of at least three actors were necessary: the physician, the hydraulic engineer, and the schoolmaster. As Bernardino Fantini pointed out, in connection with the specific origin of malaria, Grassi's equation was quite valid; but to combat the endemic disease successfully, Celli's factors were indispensable (15).

The other controversial issue, which leads directly to the issue of global health, arose out of the unsatisfactory consequences of the decision to set up control barriers to prevent the spread of exotic epidemics to Europe. As Fantini wrote, nations felt the need to "reappraise all the existing defensive strategies against epidemic disease. It was no longer enough to protect the borders of western countries or the white colonial settlements against the risks of 'invasion'" (16). In 1896 Robert Koch delivered a critical address to the German Public Health Society on the action taken to stem the spread of cholera by imposing *cordons sanitaires:* "In my opinion these international efforts are quite superfluous as the best international protection would be obtained by each State doing what we are doing, that is, to seize cholera by the throat and crush it forever" (17, quoted in 16). Only a few years later, in his hygiene lectures, Celli pointed out that ever since the first International Health Conference the aim had been "to prevent the importation of bubonic plague and cholera" caused by germs not normally present in our lands. "The dominant concepts in the epidemiology of cholera were very different from the present ones: great trust was placed in keeping cholera at a distance by closing state borders, raising quarantine barriers on land and sea that, with some states taking it literally, were extended for a period of forty days. This was all found to be perfectly useless" (18, quoted in 16).

As an illustration of how conflicting interests may converge to the benefit of health, it is interesting to note that, at the turn of the nineteenth century, many discoveries of biological agents and epidemic disease vectors were made on different continents by colonial doctors or by military scientific commissions working on behalf of colonial armies: in North Africa (by Laveran), the malaria plasmodium; in India, fleas and rats as transmitters of the plague; in Central America during the opening of the Panama canal, the *Aedes aegypti* mosquito (already reported by the Cuban Carlos Finley) as the vector of yellow fever. This research was linked to the birth of colonial medicine (which later became tropical medicine), promoted on his return to England by Patrick Manson. In India Manson had demonstrated (in 1878) the role of the mosquito *Culex pipiens* in the transmission of elephantiasis: the first proof (to be followed by many others) of the role of insects in transmitting disease. Also, this branch of the history of medicine, according to David Arnold, has been analyzed based on "the tendency to see history only in terms of the colonizers and to ignore the experience of the colonized . . . as the story of white races' achievements against a background not only of disease and hostile environments, but also of ignorance, superstition and inertia of the 'natives'" (19). There is no doubt that research on tropical diseases was stimulated not only by the thirst for knowledge but also by the effect of diseases on armies and colonists, as well as on local populations, and by the need for fresh knowledge to stabilize exploitation and extend it to the interior of continents after coastal areas had been occupied. Indeed, Arnold demonstrates that at the beginning of occupation, attempts were made to use the idea of *cordon sanitaire* to create residential niches to shelter troops and settlers from epidemics (19). And Milton Roemer adds, in connection with health care, that in Africa health services "were considered necessary only to protect Europeans . . . [they] were not extended to the African population until after the First World War" (20). In the long term, however, many others, and sometimes even entire populations, benefited both from the scientific discoveries and from the preventive measures and health care networks, in relatively short times and in relatively universal forms. From the early decades of the twentieth century, then, the protection of human health was considered a political task and an objective for the international community.

ACT II: ESTABLISHMENT OF THE RIGHT TO HEALTH

The view of health as a right arose in the twentieth century, and in the atmosphere of hope and fervor that followed the end of World War II, this right was recognized as a claim and often as reality. It was embodied in many constitutions, and in Italy with the incisive formulation of the "fundamental right of the individual and interest of the collectivity" (Article 32). The same right is defined in the constitution of the WHO, signed on April 7, 1948.

At the historical level, some have debated whether the right to health was born earlier, in the nineteenth century, as an extension of the first-generation rights, the "negative" rights of the citizen aimed at reducing abuse of power, a kind of "health citizenship" providing protection from attack by epidemic disease; or as one of the second-generation rights, social rights, according to which authorities must act not simply by refraining from creating problems but by taking positive action. In point of fact, many reasons and actors contributed to the recognition of the right to health, even before it was interpreted and validated by jurists and philosophers. According to Roy Porter, two ideas gradually emerged in the industrial countries: "that the smooth and efficient functioning of intricate producer and consumer economies required a population no less healthy than literate, skilled and law abiding; and in democracies where the workers were also voters, the ampler provision of health services became one way of preempting discontent . . . prevention was better than patching; far better to determine what made people sick in the first place and then—guided by statistics, sociology and epidemiology— take measures to build a positive health" (21). I should add that these ideas were often second best, a kind of line of retreat, after an industrial revolution that had been accompanied by uncontrolled exploitation and in the face of eugenic trends hostile to the progress of public health and health for all, based on the idea that "preventive medicine was saving the weakly with the robust and raining social suicide" (22). We must also take into account the influence of workers' trade union and political movements, which produced a dual effect: (a) the direct promotion of greater health in the workplace and a broad-based access to health services and (b) the facilitation of state policy on social security systems, by governments fearful of other revolutionary solutions. And in this case, too, divergent motives and interests acted together in a good cause. The result was not a low-profile compromise but a strong inducement to improve human life and to assign a common ethical significance to the nobly instrumental value of health.

This is the framework within which the WHO came into being. The institutions that had preceded it were set up mainly to defend rich countries of the North from diseases imported from poor countries of the South. Conversely, the proposal to establish not a bureau but a world organization came not so much from the West as from Brazil and China, with the purpose of encouraging global action and using the argument that "the weapons of science cannot be the patrimony of the developed countries alone." To this was added the idea, widespread at the time, that health was a precondition for peace, an argument that was rendered compelling by the consequences of World War II in terms of the disease, hunger, and suffering inflicted on uprooted populations and was supported by the awareness of a fresh potential to transform the need for health into a right (23). The health organization was designated "world" rather than "international" to signify that it was the result not only of an agreement among states but, above all, of a need felt by peoples; and its goal was health, not medical activities in the narrow sense. Emphasis was thus laid on the global commitment and on the notions that improvement in health was not dependent on medicine alone and that "all the factors of physical and mental improvement of individuals and peoples" must be deployed, as stated in the WHO statute. The tasks of the organization included the fight against old and new diseases and the fight for nutrition, children, vaccines and medicines, and public health (24).

The two highest achievements of the WHO, which gave the organization its prestige as a "moral subject" and an authoritative champion of global health, were truly global in their effects. The first was the anti-smallpox campaign, against a disease that in 1967 was still endemic in 31 countries and affected 10 to 15 million persons; for the first time in the history of human infections, a disease was completely eradicated. The second achievement was the Alma-Ata Conference of 1978, which, counter to the predominance of high-tech medicine, used convincing arguments and a strong moral backing to launch the centrality of primary health care. This campaign was to be extended worldwide in the form of a combination of disease prevention, adequate nutrition, clean water, child care, vaccinations, control of locally endemic diseases, suitable therapies, and essential drugs. As a result of numerous factors—including the political and ethical climate prevailing after 1945 and the attainment of independence by many nations—during the twentieth century, for the first time in history, the "eternal" scourges of humankind began to decline, levels of health began to improve, and life expectancy for the human race increased. These beneficial developments, though occurring in many different ways throughout the history and geography of the world, by substantially increasing equality among peoples, between the sexes, and among classes in the twentieth century represent an extraordinary social and biological step forward. We are all aware that the twentieth century brought us two world wars, numerous local wars, and genocide and violence. But the judgment of the British historian Toynbee is also valid, that the twentieth century will mainly be remembered not as an age of political conflict and technical inventions, but as the age in which human society dared to think that the health of the entire human species was an attainable practical objective.

ACT III: GLOBALIZATION OF THE RISKS

I am not certain, however, that the last few decades will be remembered in the same way. This impression, which I believe is widely shared, is based on grim fact: the disappointment of many hopes, the slackening access to medical progress, and the increased differences and inequalities in the level of health and security both among and within the nations. Global health indicators still point to progress, although perhaps the most pressing bioethical problem now lies in the contradiction between two phenomena: never before has the world had such healthy populations, so much knowledge, and so many possible remedies, and never have so many diseases been preventable and curable; but, at the same time, there is little will to use the knowledge and remedies in the interest of all. These two facts help explain why, although the end of the nineteenth century (after the great medical discoveries and the first results in the fight against epidemics) coincided with a wave of excessive optimism, the end of the twentieth century was characterized by doubt and even pessimism—especially after the failure of the slogan rashly launched by the WHO in the 1980s: "Health for all by the year 2000." Nor were people reassured or the WHO's credibility enhanced by its decision, when the year 2000 arrived, to launch the same slogan but extend its expiration date until 2020—then promising, "By the end of the twenty-first century"! An equally strong reason for this shift of opinion on the world's health prospects probably arises out of the perception—widespread though vague, because clouded by insensitivity, misinformation, or expectations of almost miraculous medical successes (all DNA damage cured by gene therapy, all damaged organs replaced by spare parts, and other promises of the kind)—that we are living in an age of increasing globalization of risks.

I have divided into four categories the main potential risks to individual and collective health, the diseases or the "social pathologies" that cause similar destructive consequences in human beings: (a) the reappearance of old infections and the onset of new ones; (b) the implications of environmental degradation; (c) the globalization of drugs; and (d) the prevalence of violence.

Old and New Infections

The extraordinary worldwide decline in the number of deaths due to infectious disease gave rise in recent decades to the hope of a world without epidemics. The persisting vulnerability of populations to microorganisms and viruses was unfortunately demonstrated in the 1970s and 1980s by the onset of AIDS and identification of HIV, which rapidly spread everywhere (25, 26). It was then, as Laurie Garrett wrote in a book on the risks of future plagues, that "the limits of, and imperatives for, globalization of health became obvious in a context larger than mass vaccinations and diarrhea control programs . . . the hypocrisies, cruelties, failings, and inadequacies of humanity's sacred institutions, including its medical establishment, science, organized religion, systems of justice, the United Nations, and individual government systems of all political stripes" (27, p. 10). Since HIV, a further 29 viruses and bacteria have been identified as capable of global spread, although they have so far been confined to specific areas. Diseases believed to persist in only a few countries have now been transmitted from one continent to another—cholera, for example, reappeared in Latin America after nearly a century's absence. Malaria is increasingly endemic, each year claiming millions of victims in Africa and other areas of the South, and has extended as far as Virginia in the United States. Further and more violent outbreaks of microorganisms such as *Mycobacterium tuberculosis* have been recorded, with an increase in the number of cases in both Europe and the United States (28).

The most frequent explanation for these phenomena is the exponential increase in worldwide travel. Prions, viruses, microorganisms, and parasites need no passport or visa to cross frontiers, a fact pointed out by the historian Henry Sigerist in 1943: "Now that the world has become smaller as a result of the modern means of communication . . . human solidarity in the field of health cannot be neglected with impunity." But there are additional explanations for the emergence or reappearance of many diseases. Bovine spongiform encephalopathy (BSE) spread to the human population in the United Kingdom because cattle breeders fed their livestock with the flesh, entrails, and brains of sheep, transforming herbivores into carnivores and opening the way to the interspecies transmission of prions (which thus made a "double species jump," from sheep to cattle, from cattle to humans), and because commercial interests concealed the risks and hindered prevention efforts. Tuberculosis, too, is on the increase, not only because it is an opportunistic infection that attacks the HIV-positive, but also because poverty and urban marginalization are on the increase. Food deficiencies, child labor, and indiscriminate use of antibiotic drugs have led to the selection and spread through the world of drug-resistant bacteria (29). The persistence of microbial and parasitic diseases such as malaria is a consequence of insufficient investment in research on vaccines. The amount of money available to AIDS researchers is at least ten times greater than the amount available for research on malaria, and the only explanation for this discrepancy is that AIDS can kill both rich and poor, while malaria afflicts mainly the poor.

And international travel? This is not only for tourist, cultural, or work reasons. In the past decade, 50 million men, women, and children have been forced to move from one country to another as a result of famine, social unrest, coup d'état, and war—tragedies that have always been the prologue to widespread disease. Just as human beings have tended to colonize new territories, disease-causing germs (whether bacteria, viruses, prions, or metazoa) have an evolutionary drive to colonize new hosts. As Hans Zinsser wrote in the curious but seminal book *Rats, Lice, and History*, published in 1934, "However secure and well regulated civilized life may become, bacteria, protozoa, viruses, infected fleas, lice, ticks, mosquitoes, and bedbugs will always lurk in the shadows, ready to pounce when neglect, poverty, famine, or war lets down the defense. And even in normal times they prey on the weak, the very young, and the very old, living along with us, in mysterious obscurities, awaiting their opportunities" (30). For a long time our scientific knowledge, our preventive measures, and our social policies have kept invasive parasites at bay, thus showing that the suffering they cause is not a law of nature or a divine punishment. But biosocial conditions are increasing their opportunities for growth, raising alarming ethical questions about our own responsibility.

Environmental Degradation

The last ten years have seen the growth of an environmental awareness based on the simple observation that we all live on the same planet. Health awareness has enjoyed no similar growth, nor has awareness of the relationship between environment and disease. One wonders to what extent this widespread indifference has been encouraged by the self-interested silence of those in the know, the opportunism of those with power (starting with the WHO), the complicity of the political world, and the distortions of medical science, which is extremely reluctant to admit that the origin of disease lies in the interaction between human biology, environment, and society.

But one wonders about more recent events. The picture is not totally negative. Over the past few centuries, to an increasingly profound extent, changes made in the environment by humans have helped improve human health: urban rehabilitation, for example, was decisive in the fight against the diseases transmitted by water and food, just as was increased farm production, which benefited from the use of chemicals and other products of biotechnology, in the struggle against hunger. In recent decades, however, there has been an increase in the immediate damage caused by degradation of the environment, damage that affects everybody, although to different degrees for different classes and populations. This damage is due to pollution in the air, water, soil, and subsoil and the impoverishment of natural resources, as well as to reduced quality of life in the large urban agglomerations, where the majority of the world population continues to concentrate. Many diseases originate in the globalization of unhealthy production and consumption, disease-causing factors principally distributed (unlike infectious diseases) from the developed countries and sometimes deliberately exported in the form of harmful industries or toxic waste to the poorer countries. The risks, however, are becoming global. On December 1, 1997, the *New York Times* published an appeal voiced by physicians warning against the possible effects of global warming, including:

1. Increased illness and deaths from heat waves and air pollution, particularly in urban areas, with the elderly, infants, the poor, and those with chronic heart and lung disease the most at risk.
2. Increased injuries and deaths from extreme weather events.
3. Increased outbreaks and spread of some infectious diseases carried by mosquitoes, including viral encephalitis, dengue fever, yellow fever, and malaria.
4. Increased outbreaks of some water-borne diseases such as childhood diarrheal diseases and cholera.
5. Decreased availability of drinking water due to the effects of drought, flooding, and rising seas.
6. And perhaps of greatest concern, damage to organisms on land and in the oceans that could compromise food production and alter the functioning of ecosystem services that provide the life support system for all life on this planet.

The scientists who signed the appeal explicitly acknowledged that "there are many uncertainties in these forecasts, and that some of the health effects may be less severe than anticipated." Two points, however, must be considered. The first is of a practical nature. Even when the severity of the damage is unpredictable, that there will be damage is unmistakable—and, in some cases, in the very near future. For instance, the WHO has estimated that by 2020 there will be an additional 700,000 deaths due to further exposure to particles produced by fossil fuels, and that by 2050, owing to the spread of anopheles mosquitoes well beyond the tropical zone, the risk of malaria could increase by 45 to 60 percent and the number of deaths from between 2 and 3 million to between 3.5 and 5 million per year (31, p. 126). To these ongoing processes must be added a crucial ethical question: can we avoid taking action when, although some of the developments are uncertain, it *is* certain that if nothing is done the effects will be serious, wide-spread, and irreversible?

The second consideration is of a moral nature. The consequences of environ-mental changes often appear in locations distant from the place of origin and may affect not just the living but also those yet unborn. Under these circumstance, analyses of damage and risk versus benefit are out of the question owing to the distribution of the consequences: the few accumulate the benefits; the many, the risks and damage. Even the golden rules of ethics seem inadequate, based as they are on relations with one's neighbor. We must instead rely on the "responsibility principle" proposed by Hans Jonas (32). This involves an ethics of proximity together with an ethics of distance, and thus has as its object both *the present world space* and *the time of future generations*. Jonas's responsibility principle calls for a power of prediction and prevention that can operate only on a global level, and for changes in public ethics and in the law (33, 34). Failing this, I cannot see what other approach is possible, and I would prefer to dissociate myself from the darkly ironic comment made at Geneva by John Last, the distinguished professor of epidemiology from Ottawa: "A few more dramatic disasters due to extreme weather events . . . would help to galvanize public opinion and lead to pressure for change that even the most complacent political leaders would be unable to ignore" (35). This hypothesis, as well as being somewhat inhuman, sounds like an intentional jinx.

Globalization of Drugs: Dual Circuits, Dual Standards

For the present generation, and particularly for young people, drugs are a funda-mental hazard. Drug use is often classified among the sociobehavioral pathol-ogies, together with mental diseases, unprotected sex, and violence; however, this sometimes fails to distinguish between drug use that is the result of inclination and free choice and drug use that is a consequence of persuasion or coercion. Such distinctions are important for moral evaluation and prevention. According to some, personal responsibility must be evaluated when apportioning access to treatment (for example, in cases of lung cancer due to smoking or cirrhosis of the liver due to the abuse of alcohol) and treatment should be withheld or at least excluded from public expenditure: so the argument runs, when diseases result from personal decisions or faults. Mainstream bioethics is against any such exclusion, both for reasons of principle and because the range of potentially morbid behaviors disqualifying people from treatment would be endless (why not obesity or sloth, for example?).

There is no doubt that, while drugs have accompanied human beings throughout history, abuse and addiction are the cause of serious psychophysical damage. Drugs also spawn criminal activity, often in the form of multinational organi-zations that encourage consumption and use the huge profits from the sale of drugs—after laundering the money through complicit or complacent banking systems—for reinvestment in legal economic activities and, in some cases, for political contributions in support of corruption. Many proposals aimed at reducing drug use and its attendant effects on health and security have themselves been the cause of controversy. One such plan would convert opium- and coca-processing facilities in exporting countries to the manufacture of medical or other non-illicit products. Another would establish a "damage reduction" strategy designed to accomplish two purposes. The first is to establish in the public perception a distinction between an individual's use of drugs and the criminal activities connected to drug trafficking; the second, to minimize or eliminate health risks to drug users, such as the spread of HIV through the use of infected syringes when injecting heroin. This strategy could also involve the legalization of "light drugs" and the controlled administration of heroin.

Despite their importance, I shall not dwell on these issues involving different, and often conflicting, values such as the need for individual and collective security versus the desire for solidarity with substance abusers. For such issues, practical needs, ideological prejudice, and moral trends are often difficult to reconcile (36). What I should like to emphasize instead is a kind of "double standard" that is unnoticed, or barely noticed. The United Nations has a long-established agency set up to combat drugs. It is, however, paradoxical—and explainable only in terms of existing power relations in the international community and in the control of information—that most of the alarm and action is focused on cocaine and opium and their derivatives (products certainly harmful and often lethal), drugs grown in the poor countries of the South that threaten the rich countries of the North (the U.N. International Control Program refers only to these drugs; see 37). Often overlooked are other addictive drugs—alcohol and especially tobacco—the industrial production and spread of which are the result of action by the North and the consumption of which is increasingly invading the countries of the South through the efforts of multinational corporations.

This reverse flow of drugs has aroused very few moral rebukes and almost no action; indeed, it is openly encouraged (38). The WHO journal *World Health* states that "the greatest concern for tobacco in the world today is the current increase in consumption in the less developed countries. While the tobacco market decreases by one percent per year in the West, in the South smoking increases by two percent each year. . . . Experts predict that cancer and other tobacco-related illnesses will break out in these countries before transmissible diseases have been brought under control, so that the gap separating rich and poor countries will grow even wider" (39). According to the same article, if no countermeasures are taken, estimates suggest that 10 million annual tobacco-related deaths will occur by the year 2030, with 70 percent of those deaths occurring in poor or developing countries.

Faced with these two separate drug circuits, international governments and organizations respond with a double ethical standard. The European Union, for example, has made a great fuss about its plans to invest two *million* dollars in the fight against cancer, particularly lung cancer; at the same time, it has allocated over two *billion* dollars to subsidize tobacco growing in Europe and tobacco exports to other parts of the world. As for the United States, over the last few decades it has "donated" $700 million worth of tobacco seeds to poor countries, also pledging to purchase the tobacco leaves as part of the Food for Peace aid programs. It has also threatened trade sanctions against four Asian countries reluctant to allow access to cigarettes manufactured in the United States (40). The World Trade Organization has stated that any limitations on the international sale of tobacco and cigarettes would be a serious breach of free trade rules and, indeed, it includes tobacco on the list of goods receiving priority support in opening up foreign markets, imposing sanctions on those countries in opposition. These policies have a shameful antecedent in one of the blackest episodes in the history of colonialism: the war (1840-1842) declared by England to force China, despite the opposition of its government, to import the opium produced in the British colony of India. The times and the drugs are different; the other difference in these more civilized times is merely that the gunboats have been replaced by World Trade Organization sanctions.

I shall not elaborate further on this topic, as the facts speak for themselves. But I'd like to ask three ethical questions:

1. When talking of health, human rights, and aid to underdeveloped countries, how can we overlook the powerful international organizations that (perhaps for the first time in history—at least on such a global scale), in pursuing their own interests, are actively promoting behaviors recognized as harmful and even lethal?
2. Are we supposed to think that the spread of drugs calls for attention and action only when criminal organizations are involved, and that drug trafficking deserves trade protection and penal impunity when, although their products have a more destructive global impact on human life and health, legally recognized industrial organizations are involved?
3. Lastly, what are the United Nations, the WHO, and the governments of the rich and poor countries doing to cope with these distortions and to avoid, or at least reduce, the looming massacre?

Violence in Its Various Forms

I am not going to present an analysis of the "epidemiological patterns" of violence here. I shall merely point out that they are the main cause of death in adolescents and young people, especially males, in practically every country in the world, and that they harm and destroy the physical and mental integrity, as well as the very lives, of millions of women and children. Violence is also a threat to individual security, the collective conscience, and society. Analysis of violence must take into account the fact that our century has been characterized not only by extraordinary human progress but also by war and forms of genocide that in many respects have no parallel in previous history. This modern history must help us understand that many of the roots of and reasons for individual and collective violence are to be found in intolerance and contempt for the value of life. In Colombia, for instance, this value seems to be approaching zero: in the period 1974–1995, more than 350,000 murders were committed; in 1994, murder accounted for 24 percent of deaths in the entire population (41).

It is difficult to construct a taxonomy of violence. Violence may be real or virtual; that is, the reality of violence is today reflected in (and magnified by) the violence depicted in virtual reality. Each day, each hour, violence is constantly before the eyes of both adults and children throughout the world—on television, at the cinema, on the computer screen. Analysis of violence may be based on a variety of statistics, often biased, and it is also difficult to assess whether there is now more violence than in the past. What seems certain is that we are more likely to know about it, although information is often selective and misleading, especially when the victims of the violence are women. It is mainly women who have contributed to revealing this violence, although much still remains submerged; for instance, many believe that the abnormal number of women's deaths in India attributed to "accidental fire" is actually due to the persisting use of the traditional funeral pyre (cf. Garcia Moreno, cited in 42).

A legal distinction is made between willful violence, which involves awareness of the wrongful nature of the misdeed; violence without malice aforethought, in which the harm caused is greater than intended; and unintentional violence, which is due to negligence, imprudence, inexperience, or failure to comply with laws and regulations. But is such a distinction morally justifiable? There are certain kinds of violence that under criminal law are judged to be unintentional but which are nevertheless due to a "conscious intention" in pursuit of one's own interests not to respect the rules, as is often the case for work-related diseases and accidents. In other cases, human decisions, such as to design, manufacture, and market motor vehicles with the capability of traveling at twice the highest speed allowed in any country in the world, and to create automobile advertising glorifying the driver's aggressiveness, may lead to statistically predictable increases in injuries and deaths. Road accidents currently rank ninth at the world level among the factors determining loss of "disability-adjusted life years" (DALYs), and it is estimated they will rise to third position within the next 20 years.

The World Health Organization, in considering many cases of workplace, traffic, and home accidents, has replaced the concept of bad luck with that of risk control, and the same criterion may be adopted for most of the disasters erroneously considered "natural," but which are often phenomena caused or aggravated by human negligence (43). In relations with biological science and medical practice, the first precautionary measure is to avoid the "medicalization" of these phenomena. However, medicine may be called upon for many and sometimes opposite reasons. It may occasionally even become a source of or accessory to violence. In the Soviet Union, psychiatry was used for decades as a tool of political repression, and, in Latin American military dictatorships, doctors were used as accomplices in the torture of prisoners. And reports of compulsory sterilization of the mentally retarded in Sweden and of lobotomies carried out in a number of European countries until recent times (for introducing this operation, A. C. Moniz Egas was awarded the 1949 Nobel Prize, together with W. R. Hess!) show that the application not only of the Nuremberg Code but of the Hippocratic Oath itself, "Primum non nocere," is still not universal.

Medicine is more likely to be called upon as a remedy to violence, in many cases in the form of treatment offered to perpetrators and victims of violence alike. For example, a considerable stir was caused by the decision of several judges (in some cases at the request of habitual sexual offenders) to resort to physical or chemical castration to prevent any further recurrence of the offense. The biological and behavioral sciences are increasingly looked to in attempts to account for individual inclination towards crime and aggressiveness. This line of research may lead to some breakthroughs, although I do not think that violence can be satisfactorily analyzed solely within the socio-biological category of "natural aggressiveness." Such an approach may help in individual cases or may provide a useful point of view, at least in order to avoid a purely sociological interpretation of violence, but it cannot explain the huge increases (or occasional decreases) in violence, individual as well as global, from one place or time to another. Nor can the concept of natural aggressiveness account for the increase in organized crime and in what is incorrectly (because it is neither small nor light) termed "urban microcrime." This increase has numerous causes, including—especially in the huge sprawling cities of poor countries—the contrast between visible wealth and widespread poverty. It has been said that "living in unequal societies is a risk factor not only for the relatively poor, but for individuals in other income levels, because of the higher levels of violence, and lower levels of social cohesion that affect everybody and not only the poor" (44).

It is hard to accept—whenever violence breaks out somewhere in the world, against one sex or ethnic group, against a different idea or color of skin, for ideological or nationalistic or religious reasons or to take revenge on the world, or whenever violence is manifested in the form of organized or generalized crime, or as political oppression, or as action and reaction—it is hard to accept that anyone could think: "It's not my problem." It is hard to imagine how one can feel insulated and protected, even behind a double armor of insensitivity and unresponsiveness. Just as drug addiction can be transmitted by inducing drug consumption, so violence can be transmitted, not only through the action of criminal organizations—and sometimes by the state apparatus itself—but also by material and cultural means: by imitation, by suggestion, by undue and sensational publicity, and through the tensions and strains that violence produces in individuals, social groups, and entire societies. Violence is transmitted as infectious diseases are transmitted. The difference is that there are no medicines or vaccines to control violence: it must be combated by social and cultural antibodies.

We isolate ourselves from these difficult issues in many subtle ways. In the face of violence or drug abuse, we attempt to reduce difficult facts to easy abstractions: type of act, actual or alleged cause, characteristics of perpetrator and victim. We allow ourselves almost arbitrarily to approve or reject violence that does not affect us directly, that we can neatly categorize using one or another of the stereotypes that the language of the dominant culture supplies so readily, in order never to have to confront violence as a painful reality. Any attempt at finding a comprehensive approach to the problem of violence and personal security must begin with modifying this attitude.

What Do All These Have in Common?

Infectious diseases, environmental degradation, drug abuse, and violence—the etiologies, the diffusion, the effects, and the strategies to combat the four phenomena I have briefly analyzed are different, and rarely coincide. However, they share some common features. First, individuals, classes, ethnic groups, and populations are often harmed selectively, although not exclusively, often with a severity of effect inversely proportional to wealth, education, and power, and thus introducing or reinforcing a condition of inequity. In addition, the same rule almost always applies to access to remedies—whether these consist of treatment for illness or security from violence or from possible environmental catastrophes. Against the threat of a possible rise in sea level, for example, the United States has launched the National Assessment on the Potential Consequences of Climate Variability and Change, which will study, among many other things, a plan proposing the construction of dikes to protect the 10 million inhabitants of the New York area. The 100 million individuals living in Bangladesh, at the same altitude, will have to choose between migrating and being flooded.

Second, all these threats are becoming increasingly global. There are thus new and more substantial reasons to link the immediate interests of individuals and peoples to universal ethical rights. Third, it is often possible to recognize who stands to profit from these threats that endanger so many others. I offer an example from each category: for that of infectious disease, for example, there are the cattle breeders in the United Kingdom (bovine spongiform encephalopathy); for environmental degradation, polluting industries; for drug abuse, the Medellin and Cali cartels and the tobacco multinationals; for violence, organized crime and arms manufacturers and sellers.

Fourth, and most important, infectious diseases, like pollution, drugs, and violence, have now largely become *anthropogenic;* that is, they no longer depend on nature or on chance, but on human decisions. As such, they may be modified by voluntary action dictated by need and by conscience. Risks due mainly to natural factors have been replaced by a new human condition built upon personal and collective decisions and economic, social, and cultural policies as well as upon a choice of values. The practical and ethical consequences of this explanation are quite important: if these phenomena are largely anthropogenic in nature, they are not ineluctable; they may be largely predicted, controlled, and modified.

ACT IV: THE REGRESSION OF HEALTH PARADIGMS

This globalization of risk has gone largely unchallenged, however, given the restricted or at least inadequate global commitment to prevention, to applying knowledge and resources to the search for possible solutions. This state of affairs is also due to a regression of health paradigms and to a downgrading of health itself in lists of priorities for governments and international institutions. This general tendency, although it seems to have weakened in recent years, may be seen in many fields. I shall outline the various problems briefly in the form of a short, perhaps somewhat one-sided summary of the different alternatives.

Health: Objective or Obstacle?

The former truism that health is both a foundation (as a multiplier of human resources) and a primary objective of economic development has been almost universally replaced by the opposite idea: that public health services and universal health care represent an obstacle—sometimes the main obstacle—to the growth of wealth, which is why the reduction of health expenditures has become a major imperative for so many governments. Benjamin Franklin's claim that "health is wealth" (that is, for nations) may be criticized as reducing health to a mere instrumental role with regard to wealth. Nevertheless, for about a century, this and similar propositions formed the basis of a powerful and fruitful commitment to health by governments and parliaments. Today we hear the opposite message: it is necessary to reduce expenditure on health. Public health policy is no longer decided by health ministers (created in almost every country in the mid-twentieth century) but by economics ministers. It must be added that rationalization—that is, the reduction of waste through more equitable and efficient use of resources (financial and other) earmarked for public health—is an imperative that has been neglected for too long.

From Primary Health Care to High Tech

The prevention-and-care model based on primary health care, designed to meet essential needs and to be open to all, has been replaced in most countries by a process that both reduces or eliminates public participation in the making of health policy and gives fundamental priority (even in countries with minimal resources) to expensive technologies reserved for a privileged few. As a result, while many suffer from a lack of treatment, others enjoy an excess. Although it makes sense to employ the available resources for evidence-based medicine—that is, for treatments that have proved effective—in practice, the spread of invasive medical treatments is increasing excessively. This is the case, for example, in surgery, with an excessive number of hysterectomies and caesarian deliveries. The same trend is found in "preventive medicine," where tests and diagnoses are obstinately performed even in the absence of any evidence of their usefulness or any possible remedy for the ascertained risk (45).

From Holistic Conceptions to Reductionism

In a period of useful specialization and of fragmentation of knowledge, instead of our attaining a more holistic conception of human beings and their relationship with health, the environment, and society, we have drifted towards reductionism in many different areas. For example:

1. Discussions of health matters increasingly refer to "health care systems" instead of "healthy societies" and "health systems": thus, the notion of health intervention is reduced strictly to caring for the ill; and prevention, which should include both education and action to reduce health risks everywhere, is reduced to preventive medicine—that is, to the early diagnosis of illness.
2. Often, the numerous factors affecting health are ignored except for those of individual relevance: genetic endowment and personal lifestyle. These are important factors, but certainly not to the exclusion of the many others, especially since they almost always interact with other disease-causing factors.
3. Discussions of how best to procure resources for health are focused exclusively on monetary resources, which are always described as "scarce" (without a distinction being made between absolute and relative scarcity), while human resources, potential modifications to the workplace and the environment, information, and education are neglected—health factors and intangible assets that in many cases are potentially limitless.
4. Fair distribution of resources for health care is replaced by the idea of rationing resources. The term "rationing," borrowed from the wartime period, is used in a fashion completely inappropriate in both context and proposed aims and methods. In wartime, the aim of rationing was actually inclusion—that is, equal distribution to all (with, indeed, the weaker given priority in the form of, say, larger rations) of the scarce goods available and punishment of any purchases made in breach of the rules (e.g., dealing in black markets). The aim now is to proceed by exclusion, with the decision of who is to be treated and who not determined by public heath care services, with all those who can do so free to seek treatment in the open market. This and other kinds of "rationing" already exist, in any case, in overt or covert

form: the difference is that now planners seek to extend rationing legally and to find moral justification (46).

Health Leadership: From the WHO to the World Bank, the IMF, and the WTO

The World Health Organization, although maintaining its technical and scientific prestige, has lost much of its former influence as the leader of world health policies, through its own fault and the lack of support from many governments. An analysis carried out as early as 1996 by the Hammarskjöld Foundation warned of this crisis: the WHO "is no longer the obvious lead agency for 'world health consciousness.' Critical issues such as equity and human rights in relation to health have not been actively pursued by the organization for a long time. . . . Many Southern governments view it just as one of the many donor agencies. . . . The continued biomedical paradigm that characterizes the organization is inadequate to conduct broad, intersectoral analysis of health and health problems and needs to be changed if the organization is to assume a lead role in developing and supporting creative, intersectoral solutions to pressing global health problems" (47).

Distortions such as these, combined with the growing weight of finance and banking on the international scene, have led to a shift of power and influence in this sector towards the World Bank and the International Monetary Fund (and, in some fields, the World Trade Organization). These bodies are today the reference health leaders in the world, and they contribute more than the WHO to influencing health policies—often, in the less developed countries, determining them directly. The main difference between the WHO and these other agencies is that they are certainly not "moral subjects" with responsibility for human health and life. At best, moral values are discretionary in the agencies' pursuit of their activities; at worst, situations calling for moral leadership are treated as opportunities to drain off resources towards trade and finance.

The practical consequences of this power shift are numerous. For example, the policies laid down by the WHO in the 1980s to address the overconsumption of artificial milk, which endangered the health of newborns in poor countries, were held back by appeals to the rules of free trade. An initiative designed to make available to all several hundred drugs certified as essential was hindered and thwarted. The drug registration commission was subsequently removed from the jurisdiction of the WHO and placed under the dominion of the pharmaceutical industry (48). At the scientific level, "orphan" diseases were neglected—both diseases that are very rare and diseases such as malaria and tuberculosis that, although widespread, are no longer of interest to the market because they mainly affect those too poor to buy medicines.

The increase in influence of the World Bank and the IMF became more rapid and profound after the 1993 World Development Report, significantly titled

Investing in Health (49). The domination by these organizations was clear in the years that followed, as they pressed for proposing, encouraging, or imposing "health reforms" that came to characterize health policies in the majority of countries. Although it was certainly necessary to correct the excesses of "statism," and the distortions due to the impersonal nature of public services, the keystone of the reforms was an attempt not to supplement but to replace universal health care systems with medical organizations that restricted access to treatment to those with sufficient insurance coverage or private funds. The model for these reforms, the HMO system dominant in the United States, turned out to be both the most expensive and the most unfair and ineffective system ever devised, from the point of view of both the health levels attained and the cost/benefit ratio. If we add the tendency of the WTO to include in the activities protected by free trade rules the "sale of health services" by national or multinational companies, then health, instead of being recognized as a universal right, may become a universal business—and one of the most profitable, too.

From Indivisible Health to Privileged Impunity

Lastly, the idea that health in the world is indivisible, an idea that was considered crucial for over a century and was one of the philosophical foundations of the WHO, has been replaced by the conviction, widespread in both Europe and the United States, that our populations could enjoy maximum health in isolation from the suffering of others. The same illusion about the problems and tragedies of the less fortunate has spread through the healthiest and richest social groups in all countries. I merely mention this here, although it is not difficult to find evidence in the ethical trends and practical attitudes in ourselves and in those around us. If this indifference to the inequities in life, disease, and death continues to increase, we might find increasingly difficult the mutual recognition of our fellow creatures as belonging to the same humankind.

THE FRONTIER OF EQUITY

It is in the changes outlined above that the issue of equity is situated today. Equity is an essential concern in the scenario of "global health" and in ethical evaluations in general, especially because our aversion to "unfair differences" in health generally runs deeper than our reaction to other differences (such as, for example, differences in income). The right to health cannot be defined in terms of equality, but of equity. It would be absurd—and would ignore the overwhelming significance both of unpredictable combinations of genes and of free will in the lives of individuals—to expect health to be the same for all, for men and women who are born different and who grow up in different ways. Not all health inequalities are unfair: many inequalities of health, for example, have a genetic basis. Such inequalities may become unfair, however, when preventive or therapeutic remedies are used preferentially. Inequalities due to freely chosen unhealthy or hazardous behaviors cannot be defined as unfair, although those due to induced or imposed behaviors can and should be. But there is, above all, a huge field of inequitable distribution in the number and kinds of diseases and accidents related to work and environmental conditions, to individuals' position in the social hierarchy, and to differences in knowledge and power—that is, differences related to the ways in which society is structured.

"Inequity in health," the WHO has declared, "refers to differences that are not necessary and that are avoidable; and at the same time unacceptable and unfair." Translating these evaluations into proactive terms, we may conclude that equity lies in making it possible for each individual to pursue and to attain his or her own best potential health level. This goal, while impossible to attain completely, was closely approached in the twentieth century and led, in almost all countries, to increased life expectancy. Although certainly not the only measure, life expectancy is the simplest and most revealing measure of levels of health. Despite the persistence of considerable differences in life expectancy (40 years in Sierra Leone, 80 in Japan), in the second half of the twentieth century this essential indicator showed a tendency towards convergence throughout the world, with longevity tending to increase even in the less developed countries.

Recently, however, we have seen many serious signs of a widening gap, notably because the methods of globalization are introducing large schisms and instabilities in many societies. The Asian financial crisis, for example, has left mass poverty in its wake in several countries—for example, Indonesia. The sub-Saharan African countries have been excluded from the benefits of medical progress (such as the prevention and treatment of AIDS), marginalized by the forces of globalization, and propelled by disease, hunger, and war towards demographic tragedy. A demographic disaster is also under way in Russia, owing first to the failure of a communist project based on the absence of freedom and then to the subsequent "introduction of capitalism using Bolshevik methods," as Emma Rothschild described it. For perhaps the first time in human history (except in times of war, pandemic, and famine), there has actually been a substantial increase in mortality rates among adult males in Russia—the result of disease and alcoholism and, more profoundly, of a loss of identity. Women, who generally manage to retain to some extent their role in society and their systems of relationships, suffer less; as Mark Field says, Russia is a country of strong widows.

In the developed countries, with their framework of stable economies and further improvements in "average health," the differences in health between the rich and poor tend to increase, also as a consequence of differential access to the benefits of medicine. The life expectancy of AIDS patients, for example, was short for all when no treatment existed; when drugs with some degree of effectiveness were introduced, there was a widening gap in life expectancy in favor of those with the means to procure treatment. Likewise, in Rome the waiting list for a kidney transplant for patients on dialysis is 50 percent shorter for college graduates than for those with only a primary school education. In both cases, this "artificial selection" is not based on moral rules or legal procedures; it comes about tacitly, as a result of different levels of *know-how* and also of *know-whom*—that is, of having more saints in paradise.

Whether we look at the more critical situations or at what happens "normally," it is clear that differences in health both among and within countries are growing. At a meeting held in Geneva in 1997, the situation was summed up as follows (50):

> The overall gains in health that have occurred around the world are being overshadowed by increasing disparities between rich and poor. The number of people living in absolute poverty now comprises one fifth of humanity or 1.3 billion people. In health, the gap is widening between urban and rural areas with resources concentrated in the cities. Within the same country life expectancy at birth can vary as much as by 18 years between provinces, infant mortality rates can be three times higher in a province than in another, and over 80 percent of public expenditure can go less to less than 40 percent of the population.

These widening gaps parallel imbalances in income, although the level of health and life expectancy of a population, as of individuals, is not a direct and exclusive function of either gross domestic product (GDP) or per capita income. This has an obvious biological justification. As S. Anand observed, "Unlike other goods, the purchase of which can be increased with a greater income, their importance in allowing a longer life to be 'purchased' decreases and obviously becomes zero at the extreme limit of life" (51). These gaps in health are best explained in terms of social and cultural differences and the value that individuals and societies attribute to the idea of a healthy society. In this area, "individual responsibility and social responsibility are usually inextricably intertwined" (52) and are related to moral judgments and political strategies that may or may not seek equity as a goal. In the relationship between per capita income and health, there are a number of significant variations that cannot be explained in purely economic terms. Some nations, such as Sri Lanka, Costa Rica, and Cuba (but not Brazil, South Africa, and Saudi Arabia), have a low average national income combined with high life expectancy and good health indicators. Life expectancy is 11 years longer and infant mortality is 30 per thousand lower in Sri Lanka than in other countries with a comparable income. These impressive statistics may be accounted for by the advantages enjoyed by residents of the first group of countries (Costa Rica, Sri Lanka, and Cuba) in educational level, the greater role of women in society, access to safe and plentiful drinking water, food, and hygiene in dwellings, and the degree of equity and social cohesion (52; see also 53).

Similar differences are found among developed countries and can be accounted for only in terms of the different scale of values and different health and equity strategies employed. Richard Wilkinson has demonstrated, for example, that the mortality rate is lower in countries with lower domestic income differentials and thus with lower degrees of "relative deprivation" (54). Substantial differences in health also have an adverse effect on social cohesion, while, at the opposite pole, the pursuit of better health for all consolidates cohesion and allows a stronger sense of sharing and of life lived in common.

The distribution of health throughout a society obviously differs from the distribution of other goods in several ways. One is that health cannot be acquired solely by money. Another is that health gains are often the indirect result of other changes. For example, the most important correlation for neonatal survival is not family income or access to pediatric care; more significant than these important conditions is the mother's educational level. However, the main difference between health resource distribution and the distribution of other goods lies in the fact that equity in health resources is not normally to be sought in a better distribution of existing health—that is, in zero-sum operations that take a little health away from some to give it to others. Apart from the difficulty involved in finding moral justification for, and ensuring the practical application of, such a redistribution, the opposite option—pursuing the objective of better health for all, and in this context encouraging the attainment of greater equity—acts as a multiplier of collective and individual resources and achieves the best results. These results include an increase in the quality of life and in life expectancy and demonstrable improvement in other statistical health indicators, both in domestic social relations and in the relations among the different nations and regions of the world.

WHICH GLOBALIZATION?

The question posed here pertains to the attention increasingly paid to the relationship between globalization, health, and equity, the framework within which I now discuss the ideas, values, and interests examined so far. A large-scale evaluation has been made of the risks and opportunities implicit in the process of globalization, a process accelerated by a technological and scientific revolution that has, in effect, compressed time and space in all fields and has contributed to the creation of a universal network of communications, influences, and power (e.g., 55, 56).

The claim that globalization is an undeniable necessity, a road the human species must take in the twenty-first century, has been severely criticized by many, including Vicente Navarro (57; see also 58). One of the criticisms is that globalization of the economy entails the concentration of wealth and power in the hands of a few and the predominance of international finance over all other interests. Another is that the ascendancy of the culture of globalization tends to eradicate alternatives (a widely acclaimed essay written in the early 1990s was titled "The End of Politics") and thus to downgrade the function of democracy, diversity, and free choice. Both objections are grounded on hard fact. I might also add that the market now operates in the world like a fundamentalist religion that tolerates no heresies yet at the same time holds nothing sacred, with life, health, and even parts of the human body transformed into commodities. For example, the World Bank and the IMF have often subordinated their "aid" to less developed countries to the governments of these countries, agreeing to help dismantle their systems of universal health care and welfare and install competitive insurance companies in their place (59).

Ralph Dahrendorf claims that, in the language of globalization, "competition is spelled in capital letters and solidarity in small letters"; and wherever solidarity weakens, increasing differences in levels of health result in suffering and loss of human lives. However, it must be added that in recent years there has been a rising tide of reaction to this situation and an unexpected increase and spread of health equity initiatives. Indeed, the issue is now on the agenda in discussions of health policies in many countries and at the international level.

A starting point was the birth in February 1996 of the Global Health Equity Initiative. This initiative, a result of the efforts of academics from the universities of Oxford, Harvard, Stockholm, Rome, and Johannesburg and of non-academic intellectuals from London, Dacca, and Stockholm, had the following aims: (a) to draw up a conceptual framework for health equity; (b) to develop measures and tools to evaluate equity and inequity in health research and policy; (c) to encourage empirical research in the developing countries; (d) to establish a scientific basis for the active promotion of policies and programs; and (e) to stimulate action to reduce health inequities at all levels of society by providing knowledge and projects for change. The initiative, which has been supported by the Rockefeller Foundation, has produced 13 empirical research projects involving hundreds of researchers in various areas of the world, as well as further research in "transversal" issues such as ethics, equity measurements, gender differences, resources, and policies, with the help of numerous contributors (60, 61).

At practically the same time, and quite independently, similar initiatives were undertaken by the WHO; the first, in 1997, by the World Health Forum of NGO; another at Geneva, in 1999, promoted by the WHO, Rockefeller Foundation, and Society for International Development, on the topic "Responses to Globalization: Rethinking Health and Equity" (for the contributions and an appeal for action, see 59). In addition, the main medical journals, such as the *Lancet*, the *New England Journal of Medicine*, and the *Journal of the American Medical Association*, have dedicated numerous articles, documentations, and comments to the subject of health equity. Finally, members of the World Bank and the IMF have begun discussing the topic with some insistence. This, also, is globalization.

As a researcher and participant in many initiatives, I have wondered about the reasons for this rapid acceleration of interest in health equity. There are probably two specific reasons. One is the considerable increase in inequalities in health throughout the world, documented in all investigations of the subject and obvious to and undeniable by even the most casual observer. The other lies in the response of feeling and reason to this injustice and its resultant suffering and deaths, the undeserved distress of our fellow humans. More generally, however, I believe that this accumulation of knowledge and ideas in the health field would not have been able to increase and spread so quickly without a simultaneous tendency towards change in the world's cultural and ethical atmosphere. Twenty years ago, it is true, hopes and illusions focused on the healing power of the market, which neoliberal ideology had transformed from what it had always been—namely, a strong stimulus and necessary regulator of the economy—into an all-powerful and benevolent god. But this god turned out to be cruel and capricious.

In addition to the uncertainties looming over the world economic and financial scene, one now wonders about the ethical implications of the increases in social inequality and health hazards. One wonders also whether, beyond certain limits, these increases will not multiply the difficulties of living together within and among countries. An acknowledgment of the reality of these difficulties recently came from a surprising source. I am referring to the decision adopted at the end of April 2000 by the U.S. National Security Council (NSC), a body that normally displays little concern with human health, that led President Bill Clinton to double the appropriations to combat AIDS in the African countries (e.g., 62). The justification given by the NSC for its recommendation was rather unusual, even somewhat roundabout: an NSC analysis identified 75 factors of instability in the world; concluded that the risk of revolutionary and ethnic wars, genocide, and devastating transitions of regimes was on the increase; observed that in Africa one of the major risks was the deadly AIDS pandemic; declared that these events "could jeopardize the national security and interests of the United States in the world"; and, finally, recommended that the president should therefore increase financial support for the fight against AIDS. Laudable as this unexpected recommendation was, I must point out that for years U.S. trade practice has been bitterly criticized precisely because, in order to defend patents, it has hindered the low-cost production of anti-AIDS drugs by the African countries, and that this policy has not changed.

I do not know which of the two faces of the human soul will gain ascendancy in the future—the generous or the greedy. However, I believe we may infer from the NSC's recommendation that a convergence of motives and interests may move society towards a common goal; and that in the process of globalization, the health and security of all takes on increasing importance and greater legitimacy. It is thus confirmed that the real question is not whether the increasing complexity and greater interdependence of international relations is a good or a bad thing, and whether this process ought to be encouraged or prevented, but rather: what kind of globalization, for what purposes, and led by whom? A reply was given in the *Human Development Report 1999: Globalization,* produced by the U.N. Development and Population Agency (63; see also 64):

The challenge of globalization, as the new century approaches, does not consist in halting the expansion of the global markets but in consolidating the rules and institutions that ensure a stronger governability at the local, national, regional and global level, in order to preserve the advantages of the global markets and competition but also to make sufficient room for human, community, and environmental resources, in order to ensure that globalization works to the benefit of individuals and not only in favor of profit. Globalization must incorporate:

Ethics—to reduce the number of human rights violations, not to increase them;

Equity—to reduce the differences inside and among nations, not to increase them;

Inclusion—to reduce the marginalization of individuals and countries, not to increase it;

Human security—to reduce the instability of society and the vulnerability of individuals, not to increase them;

Sustainability—to decrease environmental degradation, not to worsen it;

Development—to decrease poverty and deprivation, not to increase them.

But the successful balancing of the agenda, in the form of worthwhile "additions" proposed for the present globalization policies, is not possible without an equivalent balancing and shifting of power. As it is, power is concentrated in the hands of a small group of the most powerful countries rather than being shared throughout the international community. It is difficult to see how this power imbalance can change without making a start on the "world government" often dreamed of by philosophers, scientists, and politicians, an idea that formed the philosophical foundation, though later somewhat degraded, of the system of the United Nations and its agencies, set up after World War II. In his perpetual peace project, Immanuel Kant perceived the need for just such a world organization in order to avoid wars among nations: "A confederation of a special kind must be set up, which may be called peaceful confederation (foedus pacificum); which would be distinct from the peace treaty (pactum pacis) in that the latter aims to put an end to a war, and the former to all wars" (65).

One and a half centuries later, Albert Einstein again proposed the same solution in recognition of the need to prevent the use of nuclear weapons, with their boundless destructive power: "Is it truly inevitable that, because of our passions and inveterate habits, we are doomed to destroy one another, to the point that none of what is worth preserving will be saved? . . . I defend the idea of a world government because I am convinced that there is no other possible way of eliminating the most terrible peril that man has ever encountered" (quoted from Einstein's answer to the objections of Soviet scientists, see 66–68; on the outline of Einstein's proposal, see 69).

In the face of these dire prognostications and the events that followed, our feelings alternate between limitless admiration for these ideals and desolate dismay about the reality in which we live. However, we may be proud that the most terrible peril ever encountered by humanity has to some extent been reined in and now appears further away than at any time in the last 50 years. A certain measure of world government combined with other factors (including mutual fear) did the trick. Indeed, it did the trick in other fields as well, including some of the recent successes in the control of health hazards, in the form and with the results that I have described in Act I and Act II of this chapter.

After the migration of infectious diseases to every corner of the world, after the transition from separation to communication among the continents, another 300 years would nevertheless pass before the interdependence of all nations was acknowledged and globalization of health and security began. In the face of the common risks outlined in Act III, we cannot again wait so long, especially when the progress of many of the those risks may soon become irreversible. Globalization of health efforts is of critical importance; it is in the vital interest of all the world's populations and of those working in the fields of heath and security on behalf of those populations. If the tendency towards isolationism is not reversed, a deep conflict will arise between ethics and everyday practice. Physicians and health workers will be able to repair the predictable and preventable damage caused to human health and integrity only in a delayed and inadequate fashion. At the same time, they will find themselves with the latest technological and scientific means to effect those repairs, but operating in social conditions of diminished equity and with fewer public resources and support, and will even, in individual cases, be called upon to decide who is to live and who is to die. These fruits of isolationism will embody both an ethical abyss for the professions and activities established and developed to work in favor of all human life and a drama for those with the task of governing their community in such conditions.

The alternative is to foster global health. In this framework, the WHO should be given essentially regulatory functions, act as the "universal conscience" of medicine, cease being obsequious and submissive to international financial and trade organizations, and at the same time enter into alliances with inter-country agencies, industry, and nongovernmental organizations of appropriate prestige and influence (70; see also 43). Furthermore, information is essential, representing as it does the indispensable basis of citizens' participation. As Amartya Sen has said: "Information concerning discrimination, torture, poverty, illness, and abandonment helps coalesce the forces opposing these events by extending the opposition from the victims alone to the general public. This is possible because the people have the capacity and the willingness to react to other people's difficulties" (71). And this is especially so when solidarity goes hand in hand with the common interest.

REFERENCES

1. Berlinguer, G. The interchange of disease and health between the Old and New Worlds. *Am. J. Public Health* 82(10): 1407–1413, 1992.

2. Morse, S. S. Editorial comment: Global microbial traffic and the interchange of disease. *Am. J. Public Health* 82(10): 1326–1327, 1992.

3. de Las Casas, B. *Brevissima relazione della distruzione delle Indie.* Oscar Mondadori, Milan, 1987.

4. Crosby, W. *Lo scambio colombiano: Conseguenze biologiche e culturali del 1492.* Einaudi, Turin, 1992.

5. McNeill, W. H. *La peste nella storia: Epidemie, morbi e contagio dall'antichita all'eta contemporanea.* Einaudi, Turin, 1981 (*Plagues and People,* Anchor Press, Doubleday, New York, 1976).

6. Diamond, J. *Guns, Germs, and Steel: The Fate of Human Society.* W. W. Norton, New York, 1997.

7. Crosby, A. W. *L'imperialismo ecologico: L'espansione biologica dell'Europa,* pp. 39, 190. Laterza, Bari, 1988 (*Ecological Imperialism: The Biological Expansion of Europe,* Cambridge University Press, Cambridge, 1986).

8. Hippocrates. *Opere,* edited by Mario Vegetti. Utet, Turin, 1965.

9. Foa, A. Il nuovo e il vecchio: l'insorgere della sifilide (1494–1530). *Quaderni storici* 19: 55, April 1984.

10. Fantini, B. Pratiques sociales et médicales: une histoire des valeurs au travers des siècles. *Cahiers medico-sociaux* 40: 185–196, 1996.

11. Brambilla, E. La medicina del Settecento: dal monopolio dogmatico alla professione scientifica. In *Malattia e Medicina, Storia d'Italia, Annali 6,* edited by F. Della Peruta. Einaudi, Turin, 1984.

12. *Tre consulti, o disanime, fatte in difesa dell'innesto del vaiuolo da tre dottissimi teologi toscani viventi.* Pisa, 1763.

13. Tucci, U. Il vaiolo, tra epidemia e prevenzione. In *Malattia e Medicina, Storia d'Italia, Annali 6,* edited by F. Della Peruta, pp. 391–392. Einaudi, Turin, 1984.

14. Cipolla, C. M. *Contro un nemico invisibile: Epidemie e strutture sanitarie nell'Italia del Rinascimento.* Il Mulino, Bologna, 1986.

15. Fantini, B. The concept of specificity and the Italian contribution to the discovery of the malaria transmission cycle. In *The Malaria Challenge after One Hundred Years of Malariology,* papers from Malariology Centenary Conference, edited by M. Coluzzi and D. Bradley, pp. 39–47. Lombardo, Rome, 1999.

16. Fantini, B. La medicina tropicale: dalla medicina coloniale alla sanità internationale. Atti del Convegno di Bardolino, May 12, 1998.

17. Koch, R. Minutes of the meeting of the Deutscher Verein fur offentliche Gesundheitspflege, Madgebourg. *Berl. klin. Wschr.* 1: 31, 1894.

18. Celli, A. *Lezioni di Igiene, 1899–1900.*

19. Arnold, D. Medicine and colonialism. In *Companion Encyclopedia of the History of Medicine,* edited by W. F. Bynum and R. Porter, vol. 2, p. 1393. Routledge, London, 1993.

20. Roemer, M. I. Internationalism in medicine and public health. In *Companion Encyclopedia of the History of Medicine,* edited by W. F. Bynum and R. Porter, vol. 2, p. 1418. Routledge, London, 1993.

21. Porter, R. *The Greatest Benefit to Mankind: A Medical History of Humanity,* pp. 631, 632. W. W. Norton, New York, 1997.

22. Porter, D. Public health. In *Companion Encyclopedia of the History of Medicine,* edited by W. F. Bynum and R. Porter, vol. 2, p. 1255. Routledge, London, 1993.

23. Berlinguer, G. *Etica della salute,* 2d ed. EST, Milan, 1997.

24. Fantini, B. La santé comme droit fondamental de la personne: la création de l'organisation mondiale de la santé. *Revue Médicale de la Suisse Romande* 119: 961–966, 1999.
25. Grmek, M. D. *Histoire du Sida.* Médecine et société Payot, Paris, 1989.
26. Fee, E., and Fox, D. M. (eds.). *AIDS: The Burden of History.* University of California Press, Berkeley, 1988.
27. Garrett, L. *The Coming Plague: Newly Emerging Diseases in a World out of Balance.* Penguin Books, New York, 1995.
28. Lederberg, J., and Shope, R. (eds.). *Emerging Infections.* Institute of Medicine, Washington, D.C., 1992.
29. Farmer, P. *Infections and Inequalities: The Modern Plagues.* University of California Press, Berkeley, 1999.
30. Zinsser, H. *Rats, Lice, and History.* Little, Brown, Boston, 1934.
31. World Health Organization. *The World Health Report 1998.* Geneva, 1998.
32. Jonas, H. Il principio responsabilità. In *Un'etica per la civiltà tecnologica.* Einaudi, Turin, 1990 (*Das Prinzip Verantwortung,* Insel Verlag, Frankfurt am Main, 1979).
33. Environmental ethics. In *Encyclopedia of Bioethics,* edited by W. T. Reich, vol. 2, pp. 676–688. Simon & Schuster, New York, 1995.
34. Environmental justice. In *Encyclopedia of Applied Ethics,* edited by R. Chadwick, vol. 2, pp. 93–105. Academic Press, San Diego, 1998.
35. Last, J. Ethical Dimensions of Ecosystems Sustainability and Human Health. Paper presented at CIOMS-WHO International Conference on Ethics, Equity and the Renewal of WHO's Health-for-all Strategy, Geneva, March 12–14, 1997.
36. Berlinguer, G. *La droga fra noi: Intervista di Danielle Gattengo Mazzonis.* Editori Riuniti, Rome, 1980.
37. United Nations International Control Program. *A World without Drugs: It Is Possible.* U.N. Special Assembly, New York, June 8–10, 1998.
38. Escudero, J. C. Drogas legales, enfermedades y muerte. In *Drogas: Mejor hablar de ciertas cosas,* edited by Patricia Sorokin. Universidad de Buenos Aires, Buenos Aires, 1997.
39. World Health Organization. Tobacco alert: The tobacco epidemic—A global public health emergency. *World Health,* 1998.
40. Roemer, M., and Roemer, R. Global health, national development. *Am. J. Public Health* 80(10): 1189, 1990.
41. Franco, S. *El quinto: no matar—Comtextos explicativos de la violencia en Colombia.* TM Editores, Santa Fé de Bogotà, 1999.
42. Chen, L., and Berlinguer, G. Health Equity in a Globalizing World. In *Challenging Inequities in Health. From Ethics to Action,* edited by T. Evans, M. Whitehead, Finn Diderichsen, Abbas Bhuiya, and Meg Wirth. Oxford University Press, 2001.
43. Violence, a matter of health. *World Health* 1, January-February 1993.
44. Diderichsen, F. Measuring Causes of Inequalities in Health: An Epidemiological Perspective. Paper presented at the meeting of the Global Health Equity Initiative, China, October 1997.
45. Tombesi, M., and Caimi, V. Medicina basata sull'invadenza: La nuova inflazione medica si nasconde nella medicina preventiva. In *La salute in Italia. Rapporto 1999,* edited by M. Geddes and G. Berlinguer, pp. 45–66. Ediesse, Rome, 1999.

46. Berlinguer, G. Diritto alle cure: priorità o razionamento. *Qualità Equità* 4(16): 39–49, October-December 1999. (See also, in the same issue of *Qualità Equità,* the articles by L. Doyal and L. Doyal, Thomas Murray, A. Williams, D. Winkler, D. Callahan, J. Harris, A. Maynard, J. T. Hart, and A. Campbell.)

47. *Global Health Cooperation in the Twenty-first Century and the Role of the UN System.* Report from a consultation at Dag Hammarskjöld Foundation, Uppsala, Sweden, April 18–20, 1996.

48. Koivusalo, M., and Ollila, E. Health Policy by Default: The Changing Scene on International Health Policies. Paper presented at the World Congress of Sociology, Montreal, 1998.

49. World Bank. *World Development Report 1993: Investing in Health.* Oxford University Press, New York, 1993.

50. WHO-CIOMS. *Draft Report of Meeting on Policy-Oriented Monitoring of Equity in Health and Health Care.* Geneva, September 29–October 3,1997.

51. Anand, S. Global Health Equity: Some Issues. Paper presented at the Workshop on Global Health Equity, Harvard Center for Population and Development Studies, Cambridge, Mass., September 20, 1996.

52. Sen, A. Uguali e diversi davanti alla salute. *Keiron* 1(1): 18, 1999.

53. Sen, A. L'economia della vita e della morte. *Le Scienze* 299: 16-23, 1993.

54. Wilkinson, R. G. Health inequalities: Relative or absolute material standards? *BMJ* 312: 591–595, 1997.

55. Yach, D., and Bettcher, D. The globalization of public health. I: Threats and opportunities. *Am. J. Public Health* 88(5): 735–738, 1998.

56. Yach, D., and Bettcher, D. The globalization of public health. II: The convergence of self interest and altruism. *Am. J. Public Health* 88(5): 738–741, 1998.

57. Navarro, V. Comment: Whose globalization? *Am. J. Public Health* 88(5): 742–743, 1998.

58. Chossudovsky, M. The Globalization of Poverty and Ill-health: Assessing the IMF–World Bank Structural Adjustment Program. Paper presented at International conference Lighten the Burden of Third World Health, Cape Town, January 29–31, 1997.

59. Special issue. *Development* 42(4), December 1999.

60. Evans, T., et al. (eds.). *Challenging Inequities in Health: From Ethics to Action.* Oxford University Press, New York, 2001.

61. Navarro, V. (ed.). *The Political Economy of Social Inequalities: Consequences for Health and Quality of Life.* Baywood, Amityville, N.Y., 2000.

62. Parc, L. Sida: l'Afrique privée de medicaments. *Le Matin dimanche,* July 11, 1999.

63. U.N. Development and Population Agency. *Rapporto 1999 sullo sviluppo umano: la globalizzazione,* p. 18. Rosenberg and Sellier, Turin, 1999.

64. *Human Development Report 1999.* Oxford University Press, New York, 1999.

65. Kant, I. Per la pace perpetua: Un progetto filosofico di Immanuel Kant [1795]. In *Scritti di storia, politica e diritto,* p. 175. Laterza, Bari, 1995.

66. *New Times* (Moscow), November 26, 1947.

67. *Bulletin of Atomic Scientists.* Chicago, 1948.

68. Einstein, A. *Idee e opinioni.* Schwarz, Milan, 1957.

69. Einstein, A. Atomic war or peace. *Atlantic Monthly,* November 1995.

70. Kickbusch, I., and Quick, J. Partnership for health in the 21st Century. *Rapp. trimestr. statist. mond.* 51: 68–74,1998.
71. Sen, A. Closing address at the Global Health Equity Initiative, Dacca, December 17, 1998.

Afterword

In the Preface and in the space of five chapters I have given an account of many opinions, some disagreeing and others agreeing with my own—including those of persons and schools of thought of different tendencies. The discussions, research, and meetings in which I have participated intensely, ever since the 1980s, and to which in 1999 were added my official duties as the president of Italy's National Bioethics Committee, have helped enrich and often modify my ideas. I am also deeply indebted to Fabrizio Rufo, Elena Mancini, and other young people, who have helped me directly through their stimulating ideas and contributions.

The book is (and I say this not in order to share the responsibility with others) the result of numerous inputs, for which I am deeply grateful.

Among my friends, I must above all thank Eugenio Lecaldano. In his excellent book *Bioetica: Le scelte morali* (1) he expresses his agreement that "the use of highly sophisticated medical techniques, available almost exclusively to members of western societies," must not "make us lose sight of the fact that the major problems of justice are instead to be found on the plane of the ethical choices that involve the lives of everyone and not just of those who are in very special, extreme, or privileged conditions." At the same time, he correctly states that it is precisely by reflecting on the special cases "that we can undertake an ethically decisive reflection, namely that of the links between ethical principles with which it is considered that bioethical issues should be addressed and the principles to which we believe we must adhere in our life in general." To another friend, Maurizio Mori, a pioneer of lay bioethics in Italy, with whom I agree and disagree in more or less equal proportions, I am indebted for much encouragement and a flattering but rash comparison between Daniel Callahan's bioethical undertaking and my own (2). Callahan, according to Mori, began by exploring different points of view, and in his book, *False Hopes,* "after a long journey through the bioethics maze he ended by focusing his attention on everyday bioethics, placing the question of the nature of medicine in the foreground" (3). I followed a different path, Mori says, starting instead from the relations between health and society but, after traveling in different, independent directions, reaching similar bioethical conclusions. I think Mori's reconstruction of the paths followed, at least as far as I am concerned, is essentially correct: readers will be able to detect traces of this here and there in the book—for example, in Chapter 1, in which I deal with questions of equity regarding abortion and the yet to be born. A contribution to extending the bioethical horizon of everyday life came also from my demographer friends, in particular Graziella Caselli and Eugenio Sonnino, who encouraged me to develop the ethical issues related to population policies (4), which now make up Chapter 2 of the book.

In other fields, I must express my gratitude to old and new friends in other countries, friends with whom I was able to enjoy more frequent contacts during the 1990s after the reduction of my operational political commitments in Italy. For instance, I had long been concerned with occupational health and social analysis, but the proposal to address its ethical dimension came from Vicente Navarro, a close friend who lectures in Baltimore and Barcelona and whose *International Journal of Health Services* published the draft version of what was to become Chapter 3 of the present book (5). Among the readings undertaken at the time of writing this book, I was impressed by the foresight of Thomas H. Murray, who as early as 1983 had warned against the risk that a knowledge of the genetic make-up of the individual could lead to the temptation to select workers on the basis of that knowledge (6; Murray is now president of the Hastings Center). As a result of our meetings, I came to agree about the ethical importance in industrial relations of reducing the imbalance of power and knowledge between employees and enterprises in order to affirm the principle of justice. The stimulus for Chapter 4, in which I compare views justifying slavery with those justifying the technological biomarket, and which is more diachronic than the other chapters, came from an invitation by John Woodward and Bernardino Fantini, the president of the European Association for the History of Medicine and Health, to give the tradi- tional "Evening Lecture" at the association's congress in 1997. (This is a lighter version of the "Magisterial Readings" so prone to abuse in congress programs in Italy, especially because the lateness of the hour suggests that those present are likely to doze off during the lecture.) The discussion that followed the lecture was, despite the hour, quite lively and extremely valuable for the further study of the topic.

In order to finish recounting the path followed in writing this book and to set it in its proper time context, I must again mention that, in the mid-1990s, there was a lively reintroduction of the international ethical debate on the long-dormant issue of equity in health, now evaluated within the framework of globalization. I had been aware of the relationship between health and social inequity in my research ever since my degree thesis, written on the topic of differences in general and infant mortality due to factors related to work, education, and residence in the city of Rome (for a shorter version, see 7). It is probably as a result of my seniority in the field (now reaching half a century) that I was included in the promoting group of the Global Equity in Health Initiative, launched in 1996 at the Bellagio center of the Rockefeller Foundation. This initiative was further developed later, through empirical investigations in many countries and through numerous workshops on the ethical aspects of equity carried out in 1999 under the leadership of Amartya

Sen at the Center for Population and Development Studies at Harvard. (Numerous *in itinere* contributions by American philosophers to these workshops have been published in the *Working Paper Series* of the Harvard center.) Sen's observations, and discussions with Sudhir Anand, Abbas Bhuiya, Lincoln Chen, Goran Dalhgren, Finn Diderichsen, Tim Evans, Fabienne Peter, and Margaret Whitehead, were of great help to my work on global health (Chapter 5). Added to this experience was participation in various meetings promoted at Geneva—after the World Health Organization had reawakened from its lethargy concerning the relationship between health, equity, and globalization—by the WHO, the CIOMS, the World Health Forum, and the Society for International Development.

Chapter 5, the "prologue" to which sums up an investigation I made in 1992 of the exchange of health and disease between the old and new worlds (the occasion was provided by the International Congress on Historical Sciences in Madrid, which commemorated the fifth centenary of the discovery/conquest of America), underwent numerous successive revisions as a result of the advice, criticism, and experiences of the many persons who ultimately ventured into this field. The first draft was presented in spring 1998, in Siena, at the annual meeting of the Aquinas Foundation, chaired by Denis Szabo (Montreal), and at the University of Brasilia, at the invitation of my friend and colleague Volnei Garrafa, as the opening lecture for the academic year at the Faculty of Health Sciences. In the two years that followed, I discussed and re-elaborated the topic in many different forms, incorporating opinions, reading the increasingly numerous articles published on the subject, and adding documentation of pertinent facts and controversial issues, until the threshold of saturation was reached. I am not sure whether, in the end, the original work was improved or made worse (8).

The final judgment, of course, rests with the reader, both on this latter issue and on the whole book. Because of its complex gestation, which I felt it necessary to describe and which may have reduced the book's internal consistency and comprehensiveness, leaving wide gaps here and there (for example, there is no chapter on biotechnologies, and the topic of euthanasia is dealt with only marginally), I neglected to make an explicit investigation of the different trends in bioethical thinking and the usefulness of making a more comprehensive analysis of the relations between ethics, law, and politics—two topics I hope to develop in the future. However, this method of gestation allowed me to accept criticism and contributions while writing the book and, at the same time, to measure the growing convergence over time of ideas and proposals on bioethics. Today there is actually a common trend among many philosophers, scientists, physicians, and other specialists to tackle bioethical issues with one eye on future research and the other on the present condition of peoples all over the world. I found it highly stimulating and comforting when, in 1998, in Brazil, during a lecture tour on the topic "what is bioethics?" that I undertook with Alastair Campbell, then chairman of the International Association of Bioethics, I discovered the basic agreement in the content and reasoning behind our arguments, however profound the differences in our experiences.

I was likewise pleasantly surprised (ignorance sometimes dispenses such joys) to hear from and discuss with the philosopher Daniel Wikler (now supervisor of bioethical topics at the WHO) his theory of the four phases of bioethics. According to Wikler's view, which I can sum up only inadequately, bioethics was born as a projection of medical ethics on behalf of the rights of patients. It then developed along the frontiers of biomedicine, restricting its compass to the rarities in medicine, what "happens to only a few." Then, at the end of the 1990s, bioethics endeavored to account for, on the one hand, restrictions (or "rationing") of access to medical treatment and, on the other, the idea that every form of medical technology must be pursued, however specialized or costly. However, as a result of the work of many researchers and some substantial changes of opinion, bioethics now tends to be concerned with what happens to the many—that is, with the life and well-being of whole populations, focusing especially on issues current in the developing countries. The reasons for this are many: "One is the role we played in producing their suffering. Another is the example we give when certain behaviors become the rule in the medical profession, once sanctified. However, the main reason is that in an anguishing fashion we are sharing their destiny" (9).

Two final points. One involves a very recent matter: the present chairperson of the International Association of Bioethics (IAB), Ruth Macklin, at the opening of the IAB congress in London in September 2000, stated that the task of highest priority in bioethics today is to face the issues of "growing inequity in world health" and the dramatic plight of women, particularly in Asia but also throughout other areas of the world. The other point concerns the future: the next IAB congress, to be held in Brasilia, will be chaired by Volnei Garrafa in October 2002; the theme: bioethics, power, and injustice.

The topics and trends covered in this book thus constantly re-propose the relationship between—if these two summary expressions can be used—frontier bioethics and everyday bioethics. At least in its intentions, this analysis is perhaps the main unifying thread running through the book. There are explicit references to it in, for example, Chapter 1, in the comparisons among the various forms of sterility; in Chapter 2, in the description of the historical evolution (from beckoning to genetic screening) of methods for selecting workers; and in various chapters, in the reflections on the risk that subordination of all ethical values to the laws of the market will reduce to the status of commodity—the final commodity—human beings themselves.

REFERENCES

1. Lecaldano, E. *Bioetica: Le scelte morali,* pp. 28–29. Laterza, Bari, 1999.
2. Mori, M. False speranze della medicina. *Qualità Equità* 17: 72–81, January-March 2000.

3. Callahan, D. *La medicina impossible: Le utopie e gli errori della medicina moderna.* Baldini e Castoldi, Milan, 2000 [1998].
4. Berlinguer, G., Populasione, etica ed equitá. *Genus* 53(1–2): 13–35, 1997.
5. Berlinguer, G., Falzi, G., and Figà-Talamanca, I. Ethical problems in the relationship between health and work. *Int. J. Health Serv.* 26(1): 147–171, 1996.
6. Murray, T. H. Screening workers for genetic risk. *Hastings Center Rep.* 13(1): 5–8, 1983.
7. Berlinguer, G. La mortalité dans les différents quartiers de Rome en temps de paix et en temps de guerre. Paper presented at the Congrès mondial des médecins pour l'étude des conditions actuelles de vie, Vienne, May 23–25, 1953. pp. 280–291.
8. Berlinguer, G. Globalization and global health. *Int. J. Health Serv.* 29(3): 579–595, 1999.
9. Wikler, D. Presidential address: Bioethics and social responsibility. *Bioethics* 11(3–4): 185–192, 1997.

Index